Making Sense of
Public Health Medicine

Jim Connelly
Consultant Senior Lecturer in Public Health Medicine,
Nuffield Institute for Health, University of Leeds

and

Chris Worth
Director of Public Health
Calderdale and Kirklees Health Authority

RADCLIFFE MEDICAL PRESS

Radcliffe Medical Press Ltd
18 Marcham Road, Abingdon, Oxon OX14 1AA, UK

British Library Cataloguing in Publication Data

A catalogue record for this book is available from the British Library.

ISBN 1 85775 186 8

Library of Congress Cataloging-in-Publication Data is available.

Typeset by Advance Typesetting Ltd, Oxfordshire
Printed and bound by Biddles Ltd, Guildford and King's Lynn

Contents

Preface

This book presents an introduction to modern public health seen from the perspective of practitioners of public health medicine though it is written for a wider audience. Public health is not the sole preserve of public health physicians but we believe it important to document here our view of what public health physicians might contribute to current and future health challenges. The future will see a number of changes following the election of a Labour Government in May 1997. A Minister for Public Health will oversee a review of the structure and function of public health agencies and it has been made known that tackling inequalities in health is to become the major focus of a concerted policy response. It is therefore an opportune moment to display and describe the public health response that such a focus requires. We wish to clarify four aspects of this work from the outset.

First, we have written this account based upon our values, interests and understanding. We do not suggest it is the *standard* or *approved* version of theory and practice of public health medicine. This is not a deficiency, because, if there are indeed such authorized versions of this discipline we haven't encountered them and do not expect to. Whilst this is decidedly our account of the field it is not, we believe, an especially idiosyncratic or eccentric one.

Second, we have been selective in the topics and issues covered. Our intention is to present those issues that are both central and illustrative of the development and use of a public health analysis and perspective. The topics chosen are forward looking; by this we mean that they are issues that will increasingly shape the practice of public health in the future.

Third, we have written an account that eschews detailed academic conventions regarding references to primary or secondary research to reinforce our arguments. The end notes are included for those who wish to check on our more contentious assertions of fact and for those who want to pursue individual topics. In a book of this size many linking arguments have been left out, but we have tried to allow readers to reconstruct the arguments by using the referenced sources.

Fourth, and perhaps most importantly, we attempt to display, in the way that we cover topics, *a way of thinking* about health, disease, our environment and our society. This way of thinking will typically draw upon a wide range of individual disciplines, combine insights from them, apply these insights and draw conclusions. A partial listing of source disciplines can be given: epidemiology, politics, sociology, economics, philosophy, clinical medicine, law, social policy, psychology, environmental science. This listing represents a key feature of public health medicine as its *eclecticism*; another key feature is its *pragmatism*, but this pragmatism should be, we suggest, more influenced by theory than it has been in the past. This book gives an account of modern public health that challenges the predominant view of health contained within medicine. This is important because this medical view does not, it turns out, hold the key to understanding our past improvement in health and does not contain within its explanatory resources very much power for maintaining and further improving our health in the future.

Three themes run throughout this book:

- The importance of explanation regarding the causes of health and ill-health.

- The uses of a population (public health) rather than individual level perspective.

- The application of a public health perspective to preventing disease and protecting and promoting health.

Structure of the book

Chapter 1 gives a brief account of the current work of public health medicine by sketching out its past development. The purpose of this account is to illustrate the essentially contested nature of public health practice and outline its organizational context. The historical development of the position of public health physicians is, however, an important part of understanding both the real potential and the constraints of this function. The theoretical arguments for a distinctive public health medicine practice are introduced in this chapter and are elaborated in Chapters 4 and 5. In addition, throughout this book, we present brief case studies. Their purpose is to show how the general perspectives of public health medicine are currently expressed in the day-to-day work of public health physicians. These case studies show both the current opportunities and limitations of this professional role.

Chapter 2 outlines the evidence that health has improved for reasons that largely exclude advances in clinical medicine. The purpose of this argument is to set out the ground for a public health perspective on health and disease that understands both as the outcomes of social, economic and political generative factors and causal pathways. The organic pathology of disease is the final outcome of this causal network, but locating causes within the body without taking this broader approach is to restrict the possibilities of disease control and the priorities of a health policy.

Chapter 3 continues the discussion of the explanation of disease causation by summarizing the accumulated research that connects ill-health to the social and economic position of the individual and the social organization of society. The material in Chapters 2 and 3 point the way to a realist health policy that involves social and political changes.

Chapter 4 looks at clinical medicine and examines three contemporary critiques: the sociological, economic and managerial. It is argued that each critique overstates or mistakes the problem of clinical medicine. In response, a public health medicine critique is elaborated, by synthesizing useful elements of these existing critiques. While we present a sympathetic account of clinical medicine we contend that it is still a critical account.

Chapter 5 examines and elaborates the public health medicine critique of clinical medicine in more detail, focusing on three central issues of clinical medicine: effectiveness, efficiency and the social ideology of medicine. Recommendations for a fundamental reform are made.

Chapter 6 looks at how health policy analysts have found faults with the National Health Service (NHS) and sketches out the arguments that underlie these assessments. The 1991 NHS reforms are assessed and the likely future direction of NHS restructuring is described. A defence of the NHS is outlined that identifies its founding principles as robust in the face of a sometimes capricious reforming zeal.

Chapter 7 presents arguments for a radical reform of health policy, building the arguments from material in the previous chapters of this book. This socio-political (realist) health policy is contrasted with the *Health of the Nation* approach.

Chapter 8 summarizes the main arguments of this book – the need for a realist health policy and a reform of clinical medicine – to achieve public health.

Our hope is that this book will introduce the reader to the basis for calling for a radical reform of the NHS, principally through the expansion of what should constitute a public health policy. The facts of the matter, we believe, are established and the most important are summarized in this book, but the changes required to develop this long overdue public health policy have not yet begun.

Jim Connelly
Chris Worth
August 1997

Acknowledgements

We would like to thank a number of people who commented on the ideas contained in this book. Their interest is greatly appreciated even if we continue to hold to our original opinions in many places: Sheila Adam, Eddy Beck, David Hunter, Nick Judson, Tim Lambert, Maja Lambert, Euan Robertson, Paul Roderick, Anthony Staines and Rhys Williams. Jamie Etherington steered us through the editing process and Pam Lillie and Catherine Oxley took care in typing the manuscript.

If liberals remember the counsel of equal concern, they will construct such a theory now, by pointing to the minimal grounds on which people with self respect can be expected to regard a community as their community, and to regard its future as in any sense their future. If government pushes people below the level at which they can help shape the community and draw value from it for their own lives, or if it holds out a bright future in which their own children are promised only second-class lives, then it forfeits the only premise on which its conduct might be justified.

Ronald Dworkin
'Why liberals should care about equality'
(*A Matter of Principle* (1985) OUP, Oxford)

1

What is public health medicine?

The history of public health in the UK is largely the history of changing ideas about how disease is caused and what can be done to reduce it and improve health. The British cholera epidemics of 1832–33, 1848–49 and 1854–55 were the spurs to a wide-ranging set of actions captured by the term 'sanitary reform'. This sanitary reform period saw the consolidation of a number of social movements that were united in their belief that poverty and insanitary conditions were dependent upon each other. Public health thus took on an unmistakably social and political agenda, which, however, seemed to be weakened and even lost as the nineteenth century wore on. The institutional history of public health medicine is the subject of this chapter and so we must, for the moment, leave this wider context. The connection between public health and social, economic and political factors, however, figures largely in the remainder of this book.

For present purposes, an important landmark occurred when the City of Liverpool appointed Dr William Duncan as the first Medical Officer of Health (MOH) in 1847, and other towns and cities subsequently followed this lead. The rationale and duties of the MOH were first set out in the Liverpool Sanitary Act, 1846, as follows:

And whereas the health of the population, especially of the poorer classes, is frequently induced by the prevalence of epidemical and other disorders, and the virulence and extent of such disorders, is frequently due and owing to the existence of local causes which are capable of removal but which have hitherto frequently escaped detection from the want of some experienced person to examine into and report upon them, it is expedient that power should be given to appoint a duly qualified medical practitioner for that purpose; Be it therefore, enacted, that it shall be lawful for the said Council to appoint, subject to the approval of one of her Majesty's principal Secretaries of State, a legally qualified medical practitioner, of skill and experience, to inspect and report periodically on the sanitary condition of the said borough, to ascertain the existence of diseases, more especially epidemics increasing the rates of mortality, and to point out the existence of any nuisance or other local causes which are likely to originate and maintain such diseases and injuriously affect the health of the inhabitants of the said borough, and to take cognisance of the fact, of the existence of any contagious disease and to point out the most efficacious modes for checking or preventing the spread of such diseases ...

In the Local Government Board Act, 1871, appointment of an MOH was recommended for every local district and in the following year the Public Health Act, 1872, made such appointments compulsory. These Acts did not, however, lay down specific duties for the MOH. Attempts to define these duties came from a variety of subsequent sources, all of which, in practice, were in place well before the turn of the century. Perhaps the clearest written statement came in 1910 in the Sanitary Officers (outside London) Order:

He shall inform himself, as far as practicable, respecting all influences affecting or threatening to affect injuriously the public health within the District ... He shall inquire into and ascertain by such means as are at his disposal the causes, origin and distribution of diseases within the District, and ascertain to what extent the same have depended on conditions capable of removal or mitigation.

The work of public health doctors was therefore concerned with investigating the origins and causes of disease and taking actions to prevent them. The Sanitary Officers (outside London) Regulations of 1935 added to these duties the significant duty 'and be prepared to advise the local authority on any such matter' (affecting, or likely to affect, the public health of the district). Thus the official view of the work of public health doctors was clearly in place by 1935.

The Committee of Inquiry into the Future Development of the Public Health Function

The Royal Commission of 1871 was the means of coming to terms with a number of administrative deficiencies in the fledgling Public Health Service (PHS). Its recommendations essentially were to form the basis of the PHS until 1974. The second major review of the organizational arrangements for public health were reported in 1988. The chairman of this

Committee of Inquiry, the Chief Medical Officer, Sir Donald Acheson, stated his hope that:

> [the Committee's] recommendations will improve the surveillance of the health of the nation, clarify roles and responsibilities, show how each particular skill may be brought to bear at the appropriate point in the National Health Service within the framework of general management, and taken together, will provide a structure conducive to better health for all.

The definition of public health adopted by this Committee is currently the one most favoured by public health practitioners. Public health is defined as:

> the science and art of preventing disease, prolonging life and promoting health through organised efforts of society.

The committee explicitly stated the public health responsibilities of various institutions, including central government, local authorities and regional and district levels of the National Health Service (NHS). The responsibilities of district health authorities (DHAs) were considered to be:

- to review regularly the health of the population for which they are responsible and to identify problems. To define objectives and set targets to deal with the problems in the light of national and regional guidelines

- to relate the decisions that they take about the investment of resources to their impact on health problems and objectives so identified

- to evaluate progress towards their stated objectives

- to make arrangements for the surveillance, prevention, treatment and control of communicable disease

- to give advice to and seek co-operation with other agencies and organizations in their locality to promote health,

and the tasks of public health doctors within districts were:

- to provide epidemiological advice to the District General Manager and the DHA on the setting of priorities, planning of services and evaluation of outcomes

- to develop and evaluate policy on prevention, health promotion and health education involving all those working in this field. To undertake surveillance of non-communicable disease

- to coordinate control of communicable disease
- generally to act as chief medical adviser to the authority
- to prepare an annual report on the health of the population
- to act as spokesperson for the DHA on appropriate public health matters
- to provide public health medical advice and link with local authorities, family practitioner committees, and other sectors in public health activities.

Consequently, the tasks of DHAs and public health doctors (directors of public health and consultants in public health medicine) were seen to be almost identical, with the public health doctor being the means through which the DHA's public health tasks were to be performed. The principal recommendations of this Committee of Inquiry were accepted by government and the renaissance of public health medicine seemed to be beginning.

The fall and transformation of public health medicine

'Renaissance' means a re-birth and it is used here because the practice of UK public health by doctors during the twentieth century had, in the opinion of many, become marginal and irrelevant. The Committee of Inquiry report was therefore seen as providing a rationale, a professional renewal and a framework for a re-birth of the specialty.

The basic charge against public health doctors was that throughout the twentieth century they had busied themselves with the administration of the very diverse parts of the emerging PHS and had consequently failed to develop a coherent philosophy of *public health practice*. Before the NHS was inaugurated in 1948, health services were fragmented. Medical Officers of Health (MOsH) worked in local authorities and had, from 1929, assumed the responsibility for the former poor law (now municipal) hospitals in addition to a variety of community health services (e.g. health visiting, school medical services, health services for mothers and children, health clinics, TB sanitoria and services for the treatment of venereal diseases).

Critics of the MOsH and their ways of working were found both inside and outside the medical profession. General practitioners (GPs), during the 1920s to 1940s, complained bitterly of 'encroachment' by public health doctors into what they saw as their domain, the treatment of individual patients.

Others, who drew upon the accumulating knowledge of the central role of economic and social factors in causing ill-health, condemned public health doctors for failing to develop a philosophy of practice that adequately encompassed these factors. Jane Lewis, in her book *What Price Community Medicine?* (1986) writes:

> The public health departments added to their domain without questioning what was distinctive about public health. New thinking about health as opposed to sickness, and about the determinants of both, came not so much from the public health practitioners as from privately-funded experiments, like the Peckham Health Centre; pressure groups, such as the Women's Health Inquiry and the Children's Minimum Council ...
>
> (Lewis 1988, pp. 16–17).

And apart for GPs, the criticisms of another group of doctors, academics, gathered pace during the interwar years. These academic criticisms were too diverse to represent a coherent alternative, however a dominant critique can be identified in the shape of *social medicine*.

Social medicine was seen as a distinctive development of clinical medicine, concerning itself with the range of influences that individuals and communities encounter in relation to health and disease. It was, in the view of some of its most influential proponents, concerned with a much larger set of issues than public health. The latter's traditional concerns were environmental conditions, such as sanitation, housing, water, infectious diseases and community health services. These concerns were considered to have been largely determined by the preoccupation of sanitary reformers during the nineteenth century and had been consolidated via numerous Public Health Acts. The new discipline, however, proclaimed itself as distinctive and would consider genetic, social, economic and other causes of disease and would explicitly draw upon the findings of social science. Perhaps not surprisingly, the MOsH became rather unhappy with this 'new' way of understanding health and disease. Social medicine was born within universities and showed little interest or understanding of MOsH work. The MOsH criticisms ranged from viewing social medicine as 'nothing new' to seeing in its wide-ranging concerns an absurdly empty, because over inclusive, set of preoccupations. The distancing of academics, who in the main did see something useful in social medicine, and practitioners therefore increased. This distancing was indeed one motivation, among others, for subsequent educational and professional developments such as the Todd Commission report on medical education (1968) and the Committee of Inquiry report on the public health function (1988).

The MOsH between the wars were powerful actors in local government. They had acquired, through an admittedly rather disjointed and un-planned development of the state's concern for health and welfare, a pro-fessional interest in the administration of a range of community and hospital services. Certainly they saw this PHS as a model for a coming NHS. The Second World War had shaped the public mood for such a service and it had become a question of what form the service should take rather than whether an NHS would be created.

In the event, the architects of the NHS adopted an organizational form that dismantled the PHS and left the MOH with a reduced staff and influ-ence, working still from a local authority base. Moreover, though the post-war development of social work had occurred within the local authority public health department, there was a strong lobby to end this arrangement and allow social workers greater professional autonomy within their own social services departments. This became a reality after the Seebohm Com-mittee report (1968). The role of the MOH was therefore in need of radical reassessment.

Community medicine within the NHS

The reassessment of the role of the MOH became a central issue in the 1974 reorganization of the NHS. This reorganization ended the position of MOH and created the medical specialty of community medicine. This specialty, like others, would be employed within the NHS and it was envisaged that MOsH would become specialists in community medicine. In 1972, the Faculty of Community Medicine was founded to enable the training of specialists, set standards for knowledge and competence and examine trainees in their attainment.

The faculty's view of the role of the Specialist in Community Medicine (SCM) differed from the role envisaged by the promoters and key officials who had devised and steered through the reorganization of the NHS. Whilst the faculty placed central importance on the uses of public health sciences, in particular epidemiology, in assessing the health needs of a population, advising on service development, evaluating the effectiveness and efficiency of services or treatments and promoting health, these func-tions were seen as less important to government compared with achieving change in the NHS within budget constraints. A consensus management approach formed the centrepiece of a reorganized NHS administrative struc-ture, and the SCM was seen as the mediator between the administration and the consultants, working to achieve the organizational goals of the health authority. The faculty's view, however, was heavily influenced by academics, in particular by Professor Jerry Morris. His book, *Uses of Epidemiology*, was first published in 1957 and became a profound influence on the self-understanding of public health doctors. It offered, and still offers, a coherent ground for public health practice, seeing clinical medicine as, in effect, a branch of public health.

Morris identified and discussed seven uses of epidemiology, defining the discipline as: 'The study of health and disease in populations in relation to their environment and ways of living.' These uses were:

1 The study of the *history* of the health of populations ...

2 To *diagnose the health* of the community ...

3 To study the *working of health services* ...

4 To estimate from the group experience what are the *individual risks* and chances, on average, of disease, accident and defect.

5 To *complete the clinical picture* of chronic disease, and describe its *natural history* ...

6 To *identify syndromes*

7 To *search for causes* of health and disease.

Morris viewed epidemiology as providing,

intelligence for *Public Health* services. It is the necessary basis for action by the community in promoting health, in preventing disease, and in providing medical care. Health problems are revealed and measured, and indication given where in the population preventive and therapeutic action is most urgent, and likely to be useful.

The job of the SCM, then, in the view of the faculty, was the application of epidemiology and other disciplines to enable the better functioning of the NHS and the achievement of the goals of improved health of the population. The SCM should not, in this view, be seen as a mere administrator with medical knowledge.

The introduction of general management into the NHS

To policy makers within the government the NHS continued to underperform and continued to present well-publicized deficiencies that embarrassed government politicians. Once again a 'technical fix' for the NHS was sought and the area health authority level of organization (introduced in 1974) was abolished in 1982. Consensus management then came into the firing line. The reliance on consensus between clinicians and administrators – with SCMs being seen as mediators somewhere in between – had been found by academic researchers to result in slow decision making and small or incremental rather than substantial changes in the pattern of service delivery. This 'unbusinesslike' approach was completely out of tune with the Thatcherite agenda of the 1980s and in 1983 Roy Griffiths, who was deputy chairman and managing director of J Sainsbury plc (a large chain of supermarkets) produced his report into the management requirements of the NHS. This report, in the form of a 24-page letter to the Secretary of State for Health, was a radical challenge to established relationships. Regarding management influence on the NHS, the Griffiths Inquiry reported that:

> ... it appears to us that consensus management can lead to lowest common denominator decisions and to long delays in the management process ... In short, if Florence Nightingale were carrying her lamp through the corridors of the NHS today, she would almost certainly be searching for the people in charge

> (NHS Management Inquiry 1983, pp. 17, 22).

The inquiry recommended the abolition of consensus management and the appointment of general managers at regional, district and hospital (unit) levels. In abolishing consensus management it was officially recognized that the SCM would thereby lose some of his or her *raison d'être*, for if management would now be more directive then why bother with the 'diplomatic' management style exerted by the SCM? General management was introduced into the NHS in 1984 and the SCM's position and role again became precarious. The Committee of Inquiry into the Public Health Function (known as the Acheson Inquiry) therefore came at a time when it was widely welcomed by community medicine practitioners.

We have already referred to the principal findings of the Acheson Inquiry; another recommendation that was readily adopted, concerned the name for public health doctors – who had, it will be recalled, been renamed

Community Medicine Specialists in 1974. The Inquiry thought it would be better to rename them again as Consultants in Public Health Medicine. This new title has, so far, been found to be acceptable and the recognition of consultant status for the specialty was especially welcomed by those who had hitherto only been a 'specialist'.

Does the story end here? To many readers it will perhaps seem that after a 'glorious' beginning in the nineteenth century, public health doctors had failed to develop a coherent philosophy of practice during the twentieth century and had become a 'problem' for planners and administrators/ managers of the NHS. This account, however, is not fair to the many visionary practitioners of public health who have pushed for greater recognition and funding of preventive services, environmental hygiene and responsive health services. A fairer reading of the history would find that public health doctors have never been given the resources needed to fulfil their advisor, specialist and manager roles, and, as will become apparent as this book proceeds, the institutional basis for the authority of public health physicians (the NHS since 1974) has not afforded them the necessary scope for many fundamental tasks.

The NHS reforms and public health medicine

The introduction of general management did nothing to defuse the NHS's scope for producing politically embarrassing situations for the government. Moreover, during the 1980s the NHS had come to represent something of an institutional anomaly to those, including many Cabinet members and the Prime Minister, imbued with the neo-liberal philosophy of right-wing think tanks such as the Institute for Economic Affairs, the Adam Smith Institute and the Centre for Policy Studies. The repackaging by these think tanks of neo-liberalism had been influential in the Conservative Party's onslaught on the public sector during the 1980s. When Mrs Thatcher announced a wide-ranging review of the NHS in 1989 it was therefore expected that neo-liberal ideas would be powerfully represented in the policy prescription.

This proved to be the case. The immediately identifiable architect of the NHS reforms was, however, to be an American academic, Alain Enthoven, rather than a home-grown guru. Enthoven's idea was to use market forces to improve NHS efficiency, boost responsiveness to patients (renamed 'customers' to fit into this market perspective) and enhance 'customer' choice. The White Paper *Working for Patients* (1989) described how the new NHS would be split into purchasers and providers.

Providers would be hospitals and community health services (such as community mental health care and services for people with learning disorders) who would become NHS trusts, allowed to have a large measure of autonomy in the organization of the services they offered purchasers. Purchasers were to be the DHAs. Each DHA was charged with assessing the health needs of its resident population and purchasing health care from providers by using contracts. Furthermore, GPs of a certain size (originally it was required that they had a 'list' size of at least 11 000 patients; subsequently this was reduced to 7000) were encouraged to become 'fundholders', able to use their funds to purchase a certain range of hospital services and most community health services. Later 'total purchasing' was introduced, where GP fundholders were given a budget and the authority to purchase whatever health care they deemed necessary for their patients.

The public health functions of the new DHA purchasers were reaffirmed in the Abrams Committee Inquiry (1993). The purchaser–provider split seemed to many public health doctors to offer a strengthened basis for professional practice. Others were much less sanguine, seeing the NHS reforms as yet another technical fix that would further narrow the legitimate scope of public health practice to concerns over purchasing health care. Whilst the NHS tasks – i.e. purchasing services that are effective at the least cost – were, and remain, real and important, the concentration of public health doctors on those issues rather than the determinants of health may be seen to simply replay their failure 'to develop a coherent philosophy of practice' – the central charge of critics during the twentieth century.

The content and form of a coherent practice of public health in the future will, as it has in the past, depend upon an understanding of the determinants of health and disease. The contemporary understanding of these determinants forms the subject of the next two chapters. We will also assess in Chapters 6 and 7 how far recent health policy, in particular the reformed NHS and the health strategy *The Health of the Nation*, amounts to an adequate public health policy for the twenty-first century.

Case study

What public health medicine does

The public health physician in the late 1990s may view his or her fast-changing and future role with some anxiety. Whatever the future, however, we can remain optimistic that the epidemiological values outlined by Morris and the Faculty of Public Health Medicine will remain solidly implemented in the NHS. The key recommendations of the Acheson Report (1988), with regard to health authority functions, evolved into the core function of 'new' health authorities outlined in an important NHS executive document *Managing the New NHS* (1994). These core functions include:

- evaluating the health and health care needs of the local population

- establishing a local health strategy to implement national priorities and meet local health needs with GPs, local people, providers, other statutory and non-statutory organizations

- monitoring and evaluating changes in health and the delivery of health services to ensure strategic objectives are achieved.

The position of Director of Public Health (DPH) – as recommended in the Acheson Inquiry – has increasingly become important and influential in terms of advising the health authority, local authorities and other health agencies in that district. The DPH continues to act as the bridge between local clinicians and other health professionals and the executive board. The independence of the DPH's Annual Health Report continues to be maintained. This report is a key document in identifying local health needs through epidemiological and other methodologies, it also anticipates and flags up issues on which a health authority would need to act in the future. Examples of the latter in recent years are extremely wide ranging and have ranged from reporting on the outcomes of local health strategy, to highlighting the health needs of specific population groups, e.g. homeless single people, through to advocating an exploration of the wider use of complementary therapies in the NHS.

Despite these positive developments, some problems do remain. The employers of many (but not all) public health doctors of today are the commissioners of health care, and, arguably, there has been an insufficient shift to the real determinants of health. The NHS is still dominated by the acute hospital sector and its problems, e.g. bed 'pressures', emerging (and expensive) drugs and new technologies. From this reality, real political requirements of 'corporate identity' and 'cost-effectiveness' are both key health phrases and prescriptions for behaviour, to which the public health practitioner must, perhaps with some difficulty, adhere.

The many and varied skills of the public health medical practitioner are much in demand by many health groups and agencies. It will be necessary, however, to continue to work for effective communication and endorsement of key public health values within and outside the NHS by all practitioners, including health sector managers, to ensure that public health really is *the science and art of preventing disease, prolonging life and promoting health through organized efforts of society.*

We shall examine examples of work based on this definition in subsequent case histories.

Notes

The History of English Public Health 1834–1939 by W M Frazer (London: Baillière, 1950) gives a detailed account of the 'glory years'; *What Price Community Medicine?* by Jane Lewis (Brighton: Wheatsheaf, 1986) gives a critical account of the 'decline'. The Acheson Report was published as the *Committee of Inquiry into the Future Development of the Public Health Function* (HMSO, 1988). J N Morris' *Uses of Epidemiology* (first published 1957 and reprinted) (London: E&S Livingstone, 1964) gives a very readable introduction to a way of working. A management perspective on the problems of the NHS is well described in *Just Managing: Power and Culture in the NHS* by Stephen Harrison, David J Hunter, Gordon Marnock and Christopher Pollitt (London: Macmillan, 1992). The NHS reforms are discussed by Rudolf Klein in 'Big bang health care reform – does it work?: The case of Britain's 1991 National Health Service reforms' (*The Milbank Quarterly.* 1995; **73**: 299–337) and by Chris Ham in 'Managed markets in healthcare: the UK experiment' (*Health Policy.* 1996; **35**: 279–92).

2

Why has health improved?

This chapter and the next will, we hope, supply in large part the answers to the two questions posed as chapter titles – 'Why has health improved?' and 'What determines health?' We can begin by quoting the late Thomas McKeown, Professor of Social Medicine at Birmingham University, on his doubts regarding medical effectiveness, he remarked:

> ... that if I were St Peter, admitting to Heaven on the basis of achievement on earth, I would accept on proof of identity the accident surgeons, the dentists and, with a few doubts, the obstetricians; all, it should be noted in passing, dealing mainly with healthy people. The rest I would refer to some celestial equivalent of Ellis Island, for close and prolonged inspection of their credentials.

These 'credentials' were explored closely in McKeown's Rock Carling Fellowship lecture of 1976 and published as *The Role of Medicine: Dream, Mirage, or Nemesis?* Whilst some modern commentators decry authors who begin their exposition on the reasons for improved health with McKeown, believing that though his analysis is correct, it is by now irrelevant to modern concerns, we disagree. The meaning of the arguments marshalled by McKeown still provides the clearest basis for public health and they continue to set the agenda for substantial health improvement in many of the poorest areas of the world. Furthermore, the mode of argument he used remains simple yet brilliant and original. It deserves to be told and retold.

Thomas McKeown's historical demography

Demography is the study of the forces that affect populations – births, deaths and migration. In England and Wales, the systematic registration and analysis of causes of death dates back to 1838, though records were incomplete until 1841. It is, therefore, possible to look at rates of death classified into various causes from this time onward. By doing this for the period 1841–1971, McKeown was able to show that medical treatment played almost no part in the remarkable increase in life expectancy that occurred during this period – this increase being itself the result of falling rates of death from, in particular, infectious diseases.

Life expectancy at birth for males in 1838 was 39.9 years, and for females 41.8 years. By 1900 these figures were 44.1 and 47.8, respectively, and by 1971 they were 69.6 and 75.8 years. Moreover, the decline in death rates was much greater at younger ages; death rates decreased 20 times for ages 1–14 between 1851 and 1971; 10 times for ages 15–44, but for those 55–64 the death rate only halved during this period.

McKeown begins his analysis by observing that though the death certification records go back to 1838 the population of England and Wales had trebled between 1700 and 1851, and consequently 'this left no doubt that the decline of death rate began well before 1838'. Table 2.1 shows McKeown's estimates for the reduction in mortality rates from 1700 and assumes that the death rate in 1700 was 30 per 1000 population. As can be seen, decreases in infectious diseases accounted for the majority of the observed declines.

The micro-organisms that cause infectious disease may be classified by their mode of transmission: through air, through water and/or food, and a miscellaneous 'other' group for infections that cannot be put into these categories, for example venereal diseases. Using this simple classification Table 2.2 shows the standardized death rates for particular air-borne diseases in 1848–54 and 1971, and shows the proportion of the total decline from all causes (i.e. infections plus non-infections) attributable to each airborne disease. Standardization is an arithmetical technique for eliminating changes in rates due to changes in age structure of the population. Consequently, any changes in rates after standardization cannot be due to the population growing younger or older.

Table 2.1: McKeown's estimates of mortality rate decreases

Period	Percentage of total reduction in each period	Percentage of reduction due to infections
1700 to 1848–54	33	?
1848–54 to 1901	20	92
1901 to 1971	47	73
1700 to 1971	100	

Source: McKeown T (1976) *The Role of Medicine.*

Table 2.2: Standardized death rates (per million) from air-borne diseases, England and Wales

Air-borne diseases	1848–54	1971	Percentage of reduction from all causes attributable to each disease
Tuberculosis (respiratory)	2901	13	17.5
Bronchitis, pneumonia, influenza	2239	603	9.9
Whooping cough	423	1	2.6
Measles	342	0	2.1
Scarlet fever and diphtheria	1016	0	6.2
Smallpox	263	0	1.6
Infections of ear, pharynx, larynx	75	2	0.4
Total	7259	619	40.3

Source: McKeown T (1976) *The Role of Medicine.*

Table 2.3 shows the proportion of the total decline in death rate attributable to micro-organisms classified by mode of transmission and due to other causes not attributable to micro-organisms.

As stated, the greater part (74%) of the decline in death rate is due to the decline in infectious diseases with 40% due to the decline in air-borne disease, 21% due to the decline in water- and food-borne diseases and the other category accounting for 13% of the decline. The next logical step was therefore to examine the possible reasons for these declines.

The contending theories were: (i) decline due to micro-organisms becoming less virulent and/or due to the human host becoming less susceptible; (ii) decline due to immunization and therapy; (iii) decline due to decreased exposure; and (iv) due to improvement in general health determined particularly by improved nutrition. McKeown marshals arguments to show that the most likely explanation is provided by an improvement in general health status, secondary to improved nutrition. The detail of these arguments is not reproduced here, however a brief account will demonstrate McKeown's logic.

Though there are continual adaptations between the human host and micro-organisms, it is unlikely that a decrease in virulence would occur in a large number of micro-organisms almost simultaneously. Moreover, natural selection may be one explanation for decreased susceptibility of a human

Table 2.3: Reduction of mortality, 1848–54 to 1971, England and Wales

Diseases	Percentage of reduction
Conditions attributable to micro-organisms	
1 Air-borne disease	40
2 Water- and food-borne diseases	21
3 Other conditions	13
Total	74
Conditions not attributable to micro-organisms	26
All diseases	100

Source: McKeown T (1976) *The Role of Medicine.*

population, but this occurrence would necessitate a large prior increase in death rates so that the less susceptible would thus be selected as survivors. There is no evidence that such increased death rates occurred during the eighteenth century; consequently the first explanation, adaptation, is unlikely.

The second possible explanation goes to the heart of claims made for medical treatments. Is the decline in infectious disease deaths due to immunizations and/or other medical treatments? The answer to this is worked out step-by-step for the different modes of transmission and specific diseases. For example, tuberculosis (TB) accounts for the largest reduction of the death rate from air-borne disease (see Table 2.2). Prior to the discovery and introduction of the antibiotic streptomycin in 1947 there was no effective treatment for this disease. Available treatments such as collapsing the lung (pneumothorax) and excision of parts of the lung (thoracotomy) were of little use and were perhaps harmful in this disease. The Medical Research Council (MRC) clinical trial of 1950, however, showed unequivocally that streptomycin was highly effective in reducing the death rate (case fatality rate) from TB. Immunization, the BCG, was later introduced in 1954. But as Figure 2.1 shows, these treatments only became available long after the decrease in the death rate from TB began. Moreover, though Robert Koch identified the causal micro-organism, *Mycobacterium tuberculosis*, in 1871, effective medical treatment only became available 76 years later.

To take this fundamental point further we can look at another disease. The causes of death 'bronchitis, pneumonia and influenza', cannot be separately

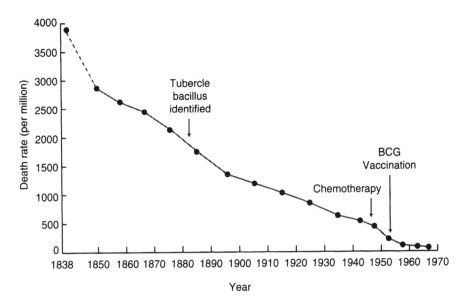

Figure 2.1 Respiratory tuberculosis: mean annual death rates (standardized to 1901 population), England and Wales.

studied as it is likely that a fair degree of misclassification had occurred in the past, confusing one disease for another. The trends in these three causes together, however, can be studied and this will correct for this classification deficiency. There were no effective treatments for any of these diseases prior to the invention and introduction of the antimicrobial sulphonamide drug, sulphapyridine, which is effective against lobar pneumonia. This drug became available in 1938. The decline in the death rate, over the whole period 1848–54 to 1971, from bronchitis, pneumonia and influenza accounted for 9.9% of the total, all cause, decline. The proportion of this 9.9% decline that occurred *after* the introduction of effective treatment in 1938 is 0.32, i.e. only one-third of the decrease.

Whooping cough was assumed (with some reservations) to also be responsive to sulphonamide introduced in 1938 and immunization had been introduced and widely used from 1952. However, the proportionate fall after these measures was only 0.10. It was by this type of reasoning that McKeown estimated that *one-quarter* of the 40% decrease in deaths from airborne diseases could be attributed to immunization or medical therapy. It should be noted that this is almost certainly an *overestimate*, since the decreasing trend prior to effective therapeutic measures has, after their introduction, been fully ascribed to the effect of the therapy.

Turning to water- and food-borne infectious diseases it is argued that medical therapy had no effect on the decline in the death rates until intravenous therapy for rehydration following diarrhoea became available in the 1930s. Cholera in Britain had always been an epidemic rather than an endemic disease, and the last epidemic occurred in 1865. This disease, therefore, contributed only a negligible amount to the recorded decline. The decline in typhoid and typhus was also due to factors other than medical therapy. Specific effective treatment for typhoid (chloramphenicol) became available only after 1950, and typhus deaths had declined rapidly during the nineteenth century, when no effective treatment was available. Therefore the observed decreases in death rates remained unexplained; they had certainly not been the result of immunizations or medical care.

The third possibility, reduced exposures, is not a viable explanation for air-borne disease. Indeed, the rapid urbanization during the nineteenth century, with its consequent overcrowding in slum housing, makes this the least likely cause for the decline. For water- and food-borne diseases, however, reduced exposure is potentially a major cause for decline. The death rates from 'cholera, diarrhoea, dysentery' accounted for 10.8% of the total decline in death rate and decreases were observed throughout the second half of the nineteenth century. These declines followed the efforts of sanitary reformers in ensuring the purification of water and safe sewage disposal. The exception was gastroenteritis in infancy, which declined only after 1900, with the provision of a safe milk supply.

The first three explanations, therefore, do not account for the observed trends, the exception being the decreases in water and food-borne diseases that followed hygienic measures introduced from the 1860s onwards. It is, therefore, the fourth explanation, increased health status due in particular to improved nutrition, that the major part of the observed trends must be attributed to.

Improved nutrition and improved health

Malnutrition and starvation are still common conditions in today's world. In 1990 more than 30% of the world's children under the age of five were underweight for their age, this proportion varied from 11% of children in Latin America to 41% in Asia. In numbers this means that in 1990 31.6 million children aged under five were underweight in Africa, 6.4 million in Latin America and 154.8 million in Asia. Malnutrition is estimated to be the underlying cause of death in 30% of all deaths in this age group. Malnutrition plus infectious diseases, such as respiratory and lung infections, dia-rrhoea and malaria, is a lethal combination and the reality in developing countries.

McKeown considered rising nutritional status to be the principal cause for the decreases in infectious diseases, mortality rates and consequent increased life expectancy observed during the nineteenth and twentieth centuries. The evidence available to him for this view was indirect since no food surveys existed. Such a survey would have had to be repeated over time and would have given direct confirmation if McKeown was correct. Still, even though some commentators disagree, it seems that McKeown's arguments, together with subsequent research, provide a coherent and persuasive defence of his nutrition explanation.

Two principal arguments are used by McKeown: first, there had been a large increase in home-grown food – enough to sustain a population that had trebled between 1700 and 1850; and second, the decrease in mortality due to infections necessitated an improvement in nutrition. Evidence of increased home production of food is both indirect and direct. The indir-ect evidence comes from estimates of the land areas under cultivation, yields per acre and data on imported and exported food. The direct evidence came later, from the first (1865) agricultural census of Britain and, from 1884 on-ward, national statistics on food production and land yield. Furthermore, there is evidence that real wage levels were increasing during the nineteenth century, so workers could afford to buy the available food (Table 2.4).

The purchasing power of these wages steadily increased during the century. For example, the purchasing power of an agricultural labourer in Sussex, in terms of the amount of wheat that could be bought in 1795, was 4.5 pecks of wheat, 5 pecks in 1821, 5.4 pecks in 1827, 6 pecks in 1836 and 9 pecks in 1851. Frazer adds that 'Towards the end of the century the standard of weekly wages (12s) in relation to the price of corn was so

Table 2.4: Wages of workers during the nineteenth century

Type of worker	1824 (s.d.)	1833 (s.d.)	1867 (s.d.)	1897 (s.d.)
London type of artisan	30.0	28.0	36.0	40.0
Provincial artisan	24.0	22.0	27.0	34.0
Town labourer	16.0	14.0	20.0	25.0
Agricultural labourer	9.6	10.6	14.0	16.0

s = shillings, d = pence

Source: quoted in: Frazer W (1950) *History of English Public Health.*

high that an agricultural labourer in this country was able to purchase 12.7 pecks of wheat, or, of course, the equivalent in other foodstuffs'.

The second argument used by McKeown draws upon the accumulated scientific evidence that the consequences of infectious disease depends largely on the previous health status of the person. This health status is itself determined by many factors, and the availability and consumption of a balanced diet which confers nutritional health remains a key factor. McKeown quotes a World Health Organization (WHO) report on nutrition and infections:

> A debilitated organism is far less resistant to attacks by invading microorganisms. Ordinary measles or diarrhoea – harmless and short-lived diseases among well fed children – are usually serious and often fatal to the chronically malnourished. Before vaccines existed, practically every child in all countries caught measles, but 300 times more deaths occurred in poorer countries than in the richer ones. The reason was not that the virus was more virulent, nor that there were fewer medical services; but that in poorly nourished communities the microbes attack a host which, because of chronic malnutrition, is less able to resist. The same happens with diarrhoea, respiratory infections, tuberculosis and many other common infections to which malnourished populations pay a heavy and unnecessary toll.

To consolidate the health gains from improved nutrition it was important that the population level did not grow faster than food supply. This, of course, echoes the argument of Thomas R Malthus (1766–1834). In his *Essay on the Principle of Population*, first published in 1798, Malthus argued that in the long run population growth would be geometrical (2, 4, 8, 16 and so on), whereas food supply would increase arithmetically (1, 2, 3 …). Hence the population would outgrow its food supply and starvation would reduce the population. McKeown points out that the birth rate declined during the nineteenth century; indeed if it had not the 1971 population of England and Wales would have been 140 million rather than 50 million. Improved living standards allowed this change in reproductive behaviour, which itself allowed the consolidation of the health gains.

The contemporary role of medicine

Whilst McKeown's argument has won widespread acceptance it is still possible that technological improvements since 1971 have resulted in modern medicine now being the main cause of improved health. This possibility, after all, is often taken for granted by newspaper headlines heralding the 'Latest Breakthrough'. Mass broadcast media's portrayals of medical life, and the way political parties swap health care statistics either to celebrate or berate health services such as the NHS shore up this view. We will discuss health sector policies in the UK in Chapters 6 and 7, but here we wish to emphasize that the increases, this century, in life expectancy related to decreases in death rates have been only marginally caused by medical treatments. Far from McKeown's argument being true but now irrelevant, it turns out that health, at least as it is measured by mortality and life expectancy, is still not determined by medical science.

A counter argument to any assertion of the marginality of medicine can start by questioning the outcomes that are measured. This argument acknowledges that death rates have only been marginally affected by modern medicine, but, it is argued, mortality rate is a crude and insensitive measure of health, well-being and quality of life. Whilst this has obvious appeal it is by no means clear that premature mortality is not an event closely related to common conceptions of ill-health, disease and poor quality of life. Death is fairly easy to measure and who, in conditions of basic need satisfaction, does not wish for more rather than less years of life? The proponent of modern medicine will quote the discovery and use of antibiotics, anaesthetics, analgesics (pain killers), modern surgical techniques for repairing accident injury, kidney transplantation, improvements in post heart-attack care and so on as unequivocally improving our chances of recovery from disease and injury and thereby alleviating pain, suffering and, in some cases, premature death. We do not disagree with this. Our argument is that these improvements are of small degree and influence compared to other determinants of health. Furthermore, to perpetuate the view of modern medicine as providing the most important way to health is to abandon a much more effective, though less discussed, viewpoint. We elaborate on this in the rest of this book.

McKeown's view (as stated in the quotation given at the start of this chapter) was that *some* medical discoveries and practices were useful in prolonging life and alleviating suffering. Surgery for accidental injury, dentistry, many maternal and childhood preventive services and, of course, the treatment of infectious diseases after the discovery of the effective drug treatments were among this group. However, he also pointed out that for many with disease, medical treatment was not able to make a substantial curative impact – those born with severe learning disabilities, severe psychiatric disorders, arthritis and those diseases where behaviour seemed to play an important role in causation: coronary heart disease and cancer. For these, and many other diseases, modern medical practice left much to be desired. Care was required, to alleviate pain and suffering rather than the perpetuation of an ultimately misguided focus on cure.

It is useful to examine a recent (1994) attempt to estimate the impact of modern medical treatment on average life expectancy. Life expectancy has increased from around 45 years to 75 years in industrial countries during this century. Preventive measures, such as screening for cervical cancer, for colorectal cancer and for hypertension (high blood pressure) would together add 10 weeks to life expectancy of a US resident. Immunizations for diphtheria, poliomyelitis, tetanus, influenza and pneumonia would together add a further 11 months. All the available evidence suggested that preventive services such as these together contributed at most two years and one month to the average life expectancy of a US resident this century.

Clinical curative services, such as treatments for heart disease, kidney failure, pneumonia, trauma, diabetes and so on, were estimated to contribute at most four years to US life expectancy. Consequently, adding preventive to curative treatments, six years and one month out of the 30 years gain in life expectancy can be attributed to modern medical treatments – that is 20%.

Though 20% of the increase in life expectancy is not negligible, it is not enough to explain the power and influence of clinical medicine in determining health policy. Explanations for medical dominance must be sought elsewhere, and we will review some important explanations later on (Chapters 4 and 5). The balance sheet of medical care shows, then, little in the life expectancy column but, arguably, makes up for this in the alleviation afforded to sufferers of depression, migraine, diabetes, asthma, cataracts, impaired hearing and trauma, among other ailments. But against these gains must be debited the reductions in quality of life due to side-effects of drugs, impaired functioning due to psychological dependence on prescribed drugs and frank disease or disability due to inappropriate medical treatment and care. What is the balance?

Let's finish by recalling the role of medicine envisioned by Thomas McKeown. In answering his own question, 'what is medicine – dream, mirage or nemesis?' he suggested that:

> ... the role of medicine should be conceived as follows: to Assist us to come safely into the world and comfortably out of it, and during life to protect the well and care for the sick and disabled.

Case study

The importance of maintaining water supplies to a community

'Water is life', so the adage goes. What happens, however, when there are threats to the supply of water? In these days of continuing serious water pollution incidents, threats of disconnection of domestic water sources and water shortages, how can we ensure that a supply is maintained and how can the public health importance of water be seen as a prime consideration?

The public health lobby has always argued from first principles that clean water is an essential public health need and a health right. During 1995, a serious drought affecting much of England led to drastic measures to conserve water supplies, including hosepipe restrictions and water pressure reductions. In the county of Yorkshire, however, the situation was so extreme that Yorkshire Water (the private company responsible for the supply of water to customers in that area) applied to government ministers for an Emergency Drought Order. If approved, a series of 24-hour rota cuts of water supplies to large populations would have occurred.

Local public health doctors led the Health Service response to this unprecedented threat to water supplies by noting publically that:

- 24-hour disruption of water supplies would lead to a higher probability of particular infectious diseases breaking out (e.g. *Shigella*, Hepatitis A) and interruption of water supplies would make control of any outbreak much more difficult

- there would be an increased risk of burns and scalds to the members of the public as a result of the need to boil water

- there would be an increased risk of contamination of stored water, which would be particularly severe for the ill and infirm being treated at home

- a potential difficulty for hospitals existed – they would be unable to discharge patients into communities which had disruption of supplies

- many health facilities, e.g. health centres, GP and dental premises would face extreme difficulty in functioning during water cut-off periods leading to potentially severe disruptions to hospital services because of increased patient admissions and access to facilities

- most seriously of all, effective maintenance of nursing and residential homes would be extremely difficult.

The above response was formulated by evaluating the available world-wide literature, using core epidemiological skills and a deal of common sense. As a result of sustained and high-profile lobbying from health agencies the enactment of the Emergency Drought Order was, fortunately, shelved. However, several areas of Yorkshire were only hours away from an un-precedented situation of planned cuts to water supplies with their dire implications.

In the longer term, the need for the protection of water supplies to maintain public health is paramount. In order for this to occur the full panoply of skills available to public health practitioners will need to be utilized. These will range from:

- encouraging public education about the need to conserve water by using the media working with local government and water companies

- working with the water industry to advise, liaise and occasionally cajole about the public health need for a reliable and constant water supply

- frequent use of health promotion techniques to advise on the appropriate use of water to prevent many infectious diseases

- working in political arenas to advocate the active use of fluoridation of water supplies as a vital public health measure in the prevention of oral disease.

The increasing variability of weather systems world-wide and the undisputed general rise in temperatures and droughts in the late 1990s led to a more serious examination of the water supply and conservation system in many countries. In all debates, the need to maintain the public's health above all else must be paramount.

Notes

Thomas McKeown's Rock Carling Lecture was published by the Nuffield Provincial Hospital Trust in 1976 as *The Role of Medicine – Dream, Mirage or Nemesis?* It was republished in 1979 by Princetown University Press. Other works by McKeown on the evidence for population growth and increased life expectancy are *The Modern Rise of Population* (London: Edward Arnold,

1976), and McKeown *et al. Population Studies* (1975) **29**: 391–422. For a view that places greater reliance on public health, especially sanitation and water purification, for achieving increased life expectancy see Szreter's article 'The importance of social intervention in Britain's mortality decline *c*1850–1914: a reinterpretation of the role of public health' (*Social History of Medicine.* 1988; **1**: 1–37). Though Szreter's work is persuasive it does not substantially alter, in our view, the substance of McKeown's analysis. John Bunker's analysis of the contribution of modern medicine to life expectancy can be found in Bunker, J *et al.*'s 'Improving health: measuring effects of medical care' (*Millbank Quarterly.* 1994; **72**: 225–8). For the continuing role of malnutrition in producing mortality see, *The World Health Report 1995* (Geneva: WHO, 1995).

3

What determines health?

The previous chapter established that increases in life expectancy in England and Wales over the last 300 years are best explained by increased standards of living. The pathway seemed to be that the increased purchasing power of workers was translated via consumption into improved nutritional status and this, in turn, conferred increased resistance to infectious diseases. Given these changes, the pattern of causes of death is also seen to change over time, with less deaths from infections but more deaths from coronary heart disease, cancers, accidents and other conditions that affect older age groups. This change in the pattern of causes of death has been called the *epidemiological transition*. This transition, in turn, produces a different age structure for the population that experiences it. Infectious diseases predominantly affect infants and children, so with the declining impact of these diseases infants and children increase their survival chances and initially represent a higher proportion of the population. If birth rate is then reduced (in part because of this increased survival) the effect, over time, is to produce a population which contains more elderly people compared to children and young people. This changed age structure is called the *demographic transition*, and the movement through this transition is found to be highly correlated to the level of economic development within a country.

Public health practitioners use epidemiology (defined in Chapter 1) to analyse the causes of disease. The starting point for epidemiology is that mortality rates (or the attack rate of any given disease) can vary, either by geographical location, over time, or with any of a number of characteristics that can distinguish one person from another. Such characteristics could be gender, age, race, social class, education, income and so on. This chapter will summarize the evidence that disease rates and, therefore, disease risk, vary in a highly predictable way with economic characteristics (such as income) and social characteristics (such as occupational social class). This evidence is now so comprehensive and systematic that the really interesting thing is that it is not better known. Getting this evidence better known must be a first priority for public health practitioners. It might then be possible to work out the policy implications of this knowledge without being diverted by the accusations of political bias that will undoubtedly be made by those who do not want change.

The first part of this chapter deals with the relationship between the economic and social conditions of a country and the health and welfare status of its inhabitants. This relationship supports and extends the ground-breaking work of McKeown and establishes a view of the 'good society', the type of society that promotes good health. The second part deals with the relationship between the individual's economic and social character-istics and his or her risk of disease. These individual-level relationships build more detail into the story and set the outlines of an objective (that is non-relativistic) account of what human beings need so that they can live healthy and fulfilling lives.

National economic and social development and health

Health is itself an area where there has been considerable debate about basic questions: What is health? Can it be measured? Is health an absolute or relative state? How does individual health relate to population health? Len Doyal and Ian Gough, in their book *A Theory of Human Need* (1991), tackle these questions and provide a persuasive set of answers. Through a detailed analysis of the concept of *need* they argue that human needs are not relative to cultural norms and can be defined and measured both for individuals and for societies. Two basic human needs are identified: the need for physical health and the need for critical autonomy. The first need may be measured in biomedical terms, that is through the absence of dis-ease, impairment or disability. The second need, critical autonomy, depends upon three key variables:

> … the level of *understanding* a person has about herself, her culture and what is expected of her as an individual within it; the *psychological capacity* she has to formulate options for herself; and the objective *opportunities* enabling her to act accordingly

> (Doyal and Gough 1991, p. 60).

The basic human needs thus provide a measure of human well-being or welfare. In a later (1994) investigation of the levels of human welfare satisfaction in different countries, Gough and Thomas were able to identify a number of independent causal factors that explain the measures of welfare they adopt. Because data on basic needs were not available for all the countries studied the measures of need satisfaction, or welfare satisfaction, used were those that were feasible rather than ideal. These proxy measures were the Physical Quality of Life Index (PQLI) and the Human Development Index (HDI). The PQLI for a country is an unweighted average of three measures: life expectancy at birth, infant mortality rate and literacy rate. The HDI combines: life expectancy at birth, a weighted average of adult literacy and mean years of schooling and a formula that uses per capita income but weights it to reflect diminishing returns to income.

One means of finding out whether one factor (say PQLI) is influenced by another factor (say the form of government) is to calculate their *correlation*. This can vary between 1 (perfect positive correlation) to –1 (perfect negative correlation). A value of 0 would mean that there was no relationship between the factors. The correlation between PQLI and HDI is 0.9742, which shows that they more-or-less measure the same thing, so we can concentrate on the PQLI in describing Gough and Thomas' findings.

There are very high and statistically significant correlations between PQLI and a number of measures of economic development, indicating that there are relationships between these factors. The logarithm of gross domestic product (GDP) per capita, adjusted for purchasing power parity of a country, has a positive correlation of 0.8577 with PQLI. This indicates that a measure of individual wealth is related to the measure of well-being. The proportion of a country's workforce in agricultural jobs has a negative correlation of –0.8438, indicating an inverse relationship with PQLI, i.e. the greater the proportion in agricultural work the lower the measure of collective well-being. The real income of the lowest 40% of a country's population has a correlation of 0.9236, the highest correlation found. This shows that the share of income obtained by the least well off has the major role in determining the PQLI of a country.

In addition to share of income a number of other factors were found to have a significant correlation with PQLI, in accordance with a number of theoretical perspectives. Dependence of the country on other countries and debt repayments was inversely correlated with PQLI; pure capitalist or socialist countries were not associated with welfare satisfaction, mixed capitalist countries (or 'social market' countries), however, did show a significant positive association; government spending on health care and on education were both significantly and positively associated whereas military expenditure was not associated with PQLI. Both the level of human rights and level of democracy of a country were positively associated with PQLI. Finally, the level of social equality achieved by women was positively associated with PQLI. These results are very interesting and support the view that economic development is only part of the societal preconditions for the achievement of population health.

That other factors are important is further demonstrated by the findings of a study carried out in the 1980s and sponsored by the Rockefeller Foundation. Given the relationship between health indicators and economic development any 'outliers' – countries with high relative levels of health but unexpectedly low relative levels of economic development – provide interesting insights into the social determinants of health. Five outlier countries or regions were selected for detailed study: China, Costa Rica, Cuba, Kerala State in India and Sri Lanka. The study of Cuba was not fully completed. The features common to these locations were: a heavy emphasis on nutrition via state subsidies and policies; very well-developed primary education which specifically included females; better-than-average equality of income; arrangements for land reform; policy priority given to elements of primary health care, such as community participation; and accessibility of rural health facilities.

Further studies have compared Kerala State with West Bengal. The expectation of life in Kerala was 59 years for males and females, for West Bengal the figures were 49 and 51 years, respectively. Though calorie and protein intake were lower in Kerala as was GDP per head and level of sanitation with piped water, both life expectancy and infant mortality rate (urban: 40 vs 61 per 1000 live births) were better in Kerala State. The explanation lies in what might be called the degree of social integration achieved in Kerala State. This is measured by the higher level of female education (ages 6–10: 86% vs 58%; ages 11–13: 74% vs 32%) and the higher participation rate in elections (84% vs 56%).

One key determinant that has emerged in cross-national health research is female education, which deserves particular attention. Those countries that have made education of females a priority have higher life expectancies and lower infant mortality rates than countries without such policies. This relationship is independent of the level of economic development. Furthermore, it has been estimated that a 10% increase in female literacy is associated with a 10% reduction in child mortality rate. This relationship is specific for female literacy, male literacy has a negligible effect. As little as 1–3 years of maternal education is associated with a 15% reduction in child mortality rate, paternal education of this level is associated with a 6% reduction.

The relationships described above refer both to developing and developed countries, however there is an argument that after a particular level of development the relationship between per capita GDP and GNP and health indicators such as life expectancy breaks down. This is asserted by those who wish to explain the shape of the relationship between these variables. Figure 3.1 shows that after around $5000 per capita income (in 1991 international dollars) the curve appears to flatten out, so that further increases in GNP per capita produces only marginal increases in life expectancy. Furthermore, it seems that as time goes on the same level of GNP per capita is associated with and increasing level of life expectancy. How can this be explained?

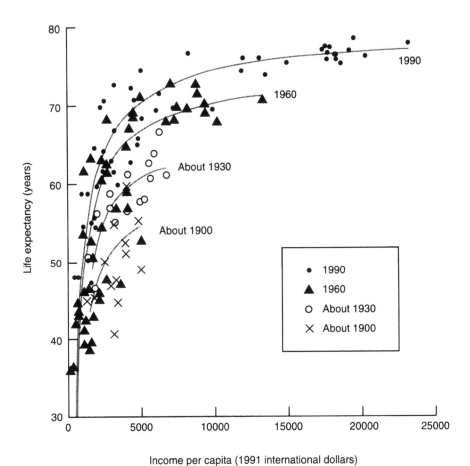

Figure 3.1 Life expectancy and income per capita for selected countries and periods. Source: World Bank, *World Development Report*, 1993.

There are a number of possible explanations for these findings. First, we should consider what GNP or GDP per capita actually measures. It does not measure how much an 'average' person in the relevant country receives in terms of purchasing power for goods and services. It should, therefore, come as no surprise that better measures of income distribution re-establish the linear relationship between income and life expectancy at birth. What matters is not the national wealth but the personal wealth of individuals or (given certain circumstances) households.

Another explanation for the plateau region of Figure 3.1 is to invoke a thoroughgoing relativism. This is implied by the observed linearity of the relationship between the logarithm of GNP per capita and life expectancy. In this case a given proportionate increase in GNP per capita is associated with a given absolute increase in life expectancy: doubling of GNP per capita from (say) $1000 to $2000 will produce the same increase as a doubling of GNP per capita from $5000 to $10 000. We will see later that within a country higher income is associated with higher life expectancy yet this close relationship is not reflected in the plateau region of the relationship between countries. The explanation, it is claimed, is that within countries it is still the relative income not the absolute income that determines health status.

This is not the place to decide between these two explanations except to point out that distribution of income is a central issue in both. In the first, certain distribution measures simply provide a better measure of what is really required, i.e. individual income; in the second explanation a case is being made for more equal income distributions as in themselves being the significant variable.

The second feature of Figure 3.1 is the increase in life expectancy 'bought' by the same level of GNP per capita as time goes by. It seems to us that Richard Wilkinson has provided an elegant explanation of this. He suggests that attention must be given to the *quality* of produced goods and services rather than just their *quantity*. Over time the quality of goods and services will increase even as their price (adjusted for inflation) may actually fall. This phenomenon is well recognized in high-technology consumer goods and in other markets, for example foodstuffs. This observation has great importance for those who argue that modern societies are consuming too many resources and are, in the process, producing environmental degradation and pollution. *Zero growth, it appears, yields around three years extra life expectancy per decade.*

Individual social and economic status and health

The relationship between poverty and health has long been recognized, finding systematic expression first (though arguably) in the Leeds surgeon Charles Turner Thackrah's book *The Effects of Arts, Trades and Professions on Health and Longevity*, published in 1831–2. The exposure of men, women and children to dangerous dusts, machinery, chemicals and filthy overcrowded workshops is clearly described and these conditions are related as causes of illness, disease, disability and premature death. Later, both Edwin Chadwick and Friedrich Engels, among others, published influential accounts of the appalling working and living conditions to be found in industrial towns and cities – these conditions being in stark contrast with those enjoyed by the affluent owners of the mills and factories. Dr William Farr, working at the Registrar General's office, initiated in the 1870s the publication of Decennial Supplements, which related death rates to occupations, giving a clear statistical credibility to the influence of occupational conditions on risk of death and life expectancy.

Extending this understanding to life outside factories, however, was not straightforward. The Victorian understanding of such matters may be summed up in the formula *disease causes poverty*. This inversion of our contemporary view had a number of advantages. Sanitary reform could be seen as a legitimate and *scientific* means for eradicating or reducing both disease and poverty. Attacking poverty itself was not a political or even moral option for a country that had long seen it as right to draw distinctions between 'honest' poverty and 'dangerous', 'parasitic' pauperism. Paupers were, it was widely held, to blame for their own circumstances and it would have been both foolish and immoral to the Victorians to alleviate their poverty by local or government action.

The announcement of the discovery of the tuberculosis bacillus in 1872 heralded the development of the science of bacteriology. From this time onwards the vision of sanitary reform would narrow, abolish the germ, it was said, and disease would be abolished. Working and living conditions would henceforth become secondary concerns, increasingly seen as part of a political rather than a health agenda.

The rediscovery of poverty or, more broadly, deprivation, as a cause of disease emerged simultaneously in the UK and the USA. This work had to wait until the early part of the twentieth century and followed the collection of health data that could be analysed by using poverty or deprivation measures. These data enabled researchers to discern striking regularities in the patterns that emerged.

The 'measures of poverty' adopted in the UK and the USA differed. In the UK, a system of social classes based upon the perceived social ranking (or status) of occupations was devised in 1911 (see Box 3.1); in the USA poverty was measured by either the years of education and the level of education acquired or the income earned by an individual. Edgar Sydenstricker, who was the US Public Health Service's first statistician, produced innovative measures such as the 'fammain' to be used in studies of deprivation and health. The fammain stood for 'food expense for adult male maintenance' thus relating income to its ability to purchase an adequate amount (1 fammain) of food, other people were able to be assigned adequate food intakes in terms of this measure, e.g. an adult female was assigned 0.8.

Numerous studies relating poor health to low income or, in the UK, lower social class, were published in the first half of the twentieth century. In the USA the Cold War made official agencies wary about articulating the findings of these studies and for a period substantive research ceased. In the UK the 1970s saw the start of what was to become the classic research statement on deprivation and health. This statement was published in 1980 as the *Report of the Working Group on Inequalities in Health*, more briefly known as the *Black Report* after its chairman, Sir Douglas Black.

The Working Group was set up in 1977 by David Ennals, then Labour Secretary of State for Social Services, and it completed its work in 1980. The report of the Group was delivered in April 1980 to Patrick Jenkin, the Secretary of State of the newly elected Conservative Government. Rather than publishing the report in the usual way only 260 cyclostyled copies were made available, no press release or press conference was arranged and only a few copies were sent to journalists on the Friday before the August Bank Holiday. Even though Sir Douglas Black was told not to give a press conference he defied this and held one at the Royal College of Physicians'

Box 3.1: Occupational social class

I   Professional (for example, accountant, doctor, lawyer)
II   Intermediate (for example, manager, nurse, school teacher)
IIIN   Skilled non-manual (for example, clerical worker, secretary, shop assistant)
IIIM   Skilled manual (for example, bus driver, butcher, carpenter, coal-face worker)
IV   Partly skilled (for example, agricultural worker, bus conductor, postman)
V   Unskilled (for example, cleaner, dock worker, labourer)

building in Regent's Park. The general and medical press took up the report, and reported its publication circumstances, ensuring that it achieved, contrary to government intentions, a wide public impact.

The Foreword to the report was written by Patrick Jenkin who made it clear that he understood the report's argument. He wrote:

> It will be seen that the Group has reached the view that the causes of health inequalities are so deep-rooted that only a major and wide-ranging programme of public expenditure is capable of altering the pattern.

He, however, continued:

> I must make it clear that additional expenditure on the scale which could result from the report's recommendations – the amount involved could be upwards of £2 billion a year – is quite unrealistic in present or any foreseeable economic circumstances, quite apart from any judgement that may be formed of the effectiveness of such expenditure in dealing with the problems identified. I cannot, therefore, endorse the Group's recommendations. I am making the report available for discussion, but without any commitment by the government to its proposals.

We need now to look at the findings that the Group produced and at their interpretation of these findings.

The Black Report

The Working Group comprised Professor Sir Douglas Black, former Chief Scientist to the Department of Health, who was then President of the Royal College of Physicians of London, Professor Jerry Morris (whom we have already met in Chapter 2), Dr Cyril Smith, Secretary of the Social Science Research Council, and Professor Peter Townsend, a sociologist from Essex University. The terms of reference of the Group were:

'1 to assemble available information about the differences in health status among the social classes and about factors which might contribute to these, including relevant data from other industrial countries

2 to analyse this material in order to identify possible causal relationships, to examine the hypotheses that have been formulated and the testing of them, and to assess the implications for policy

3 to suggest what further research should be initiated.'

The findings of the Group were clear – for the great majority of diseases there existed a social class gradient for mortality rates, with those in the higher social classes faring better than those in the lower classes. Figure 3.2 shows these findings for adult males and married women, with women classified according to their husbands' occupation. If the mortality rates are broken down by age this gradient is found to be a constant feature, more marked, however, in the early years of life compared with the start of adulthood. Children born to unskilled (social class V) families have double the risk of dying at birth or in the first month of life (neonatal mortality rate) compared with children born to professional (social class I) families. Between 1 and 14 years of age the class V/class I mortality ratio for boys

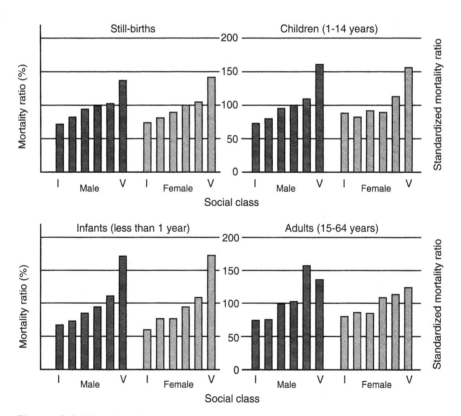

Figure 3.2 Mortality by occupational class and age. Relative mortality (%) is the ratio of rates for the occupational class to the rate for all males (or females). Source: *Occupational Mortality 1970–72*, HMSO, 1978, p. 196.

is around two, and is 1.5 to 1.9 for girls. As Figure 3.2 shows, the V/I ratios narrow during adulthood (ages 16–64) but nevertheless remain distinct.

The vertical axis of Figure 3.2 shows the 'standardized mortality ratio' (SMR), this takes account of the differing age structures of the social class groups and produces a scale where 'average death rate expectancy' for the entire population would be 100; above this is excessive and below 100 is less than expected.

Further differentials in SMR were also found, with higher SMRs for men compared with women in all social classes; similarly for those living in northern parts of Britain or in Wales compared with southern regions; and for those renting housing compared to owner-occupiers.

The Black Report used data on trends in social class SMRs up until 1969–72, these showed that post Second World War inequalities in SMRs had increased during the 1950s and 1960s. The *overall* mortality rates (all causes) had declined during this period 1949–72, however, this masked differences between the social classes – for men aged 25–44 death rates declined in all social classes over the period 1949–71. For men aged 45–54, death rates declined in social classes I and II but remained nearly static for social class IV and V. For men aged 55–64, death rates declined in classes I to III but rose in classes IV and V. For married women the spread of inequality had been (excepting women aged 25–34) narrower than for men, however, over the period 1949–71 this spread had increased. In women aged 45–54, for example, the death rate of classes IV and V, expressed as a percentage of that in classes I and II, was 133 in 1949–53 but had increased to 164 by 1970–72.

For infants, though absolute infant mortality rates (deaths under age 1 year per 1000 live births) had decreased since the 1930s, there remained stark social class inequalities in the 1970–72 data. The class V/I infant mortality rate ratio in 1930–32 was 80/32, i.e. 2.50; this ratio in 1970–72 was 31/12, i.e. 2.58. Though absolute rates had fallen in each class the ratio, a measure of the relativity of rates, had increased.

So far the social class inequalities reported have been for death rates, the Black Report expanded this to report differences in morbidity. Morbidity is a term for ill-health. Self-reported ill-health data are collected in the General Household Survey and were analysed by social class. These data showed marked inequalities with social classes IV and V reporting more 'acute sickness' and 'long-standing illness' than social class I.

Though the Black Report's findings were consistent and, taken together, unequivocally pointed to the importance of economic and social factors in determining health, they had produced an analysis that, at the time of publication, was nearly a decade out of date. To remedy this Margaret

Whitehead, in 1986, was asked by David Player, the then Director General of the Health Education Council, to update the evidence on inequalities in health and report on progress concerning the 37 recommendations made in the Black Report. This report, *The Health Divide*, was published in 1987 under similar circumstances and to similar political controversy that had attended the appearance of the Black Report.

The Health Divide showed that the analyses produced in the Black Report continued to be valid and that there had been *increases* in the social class inequalities in death rates and in self-reported ill-health. A valuable feature of *The Health Divide* was its achievement in identifying and interpreting a large number of relevant research studies on inequalities in health. For example, there had been some criticism of the data used in the Black Report regarding the ascription of deaths to social classes. This difficulty happened because the social class information that was used was gathered from the informants who would have reported and registered the deaths. Thus there might have been scope for an informant increasing or decreasing the social class of a decedent and thus biasing the data on class gradients. In 1971 the UK Office of Population Censuses and Surveys (OPCS) had started the Longitudinal Study (LS). This took a 1% sample of the population of England and Wales from the 1971 census and followed up individuals and households for registered events such as births, marriages, cancer registrations and deaths. Thus in the LS the classification of social class is based on the self-report of a living person, rather than by an informant after the subject's death. The social gradients found in the LS showed a clear two-fold difference between the higher and lower social classes with the gradient in the expected direction. Furthermore, this study shows that even after retirement age these social class gradients persist at almost the same level as for people of working age.

The LS also shows a clear gradient in mortality rates for those who are unemployed, this might have been expected because disease might itself cause unemployment. However, the LS found a significantly higher rate of death even among those who are 'seeking work', a group that would if anything be self-selected for lack of disease. Moreover, this adverse effect of unemployment persisted even after the data were adjusted for the known effects of social class. This showed an independent adverse effect of unemployment on risk of mortality from a number of diseases, such as coronary heart disease, cancer, accidents, violence and suicide.

The effects of housing conditions were also investigated in the LS and there was a clear increase in death rates in those who rented (privately or from local authority) compared with owner-occupiers. This difference was not explained by differing social class distributions.

Whitehead cites a vast amount of additional evidence which leaves the open-minded reader in no doubt regarding the consistency and validity of these research findings. We now must ask what are the possible explanations for such health inequalities?

Four explanations of inequalities in health

The Black Report identified four possible explanations for their findings. First, it might be that the findings were spurious, simply being an artefact of faulty data. It is known that there have been considerable reclassifications of occupations since the first occupational classification of 1911; moreover the proportions in various social classes have changed markedly over the years. This explanation was considered by the authors of the Black Report and, later, by Whitehead to be false. Though some misclassification of social class had undoubtedly been experienced this would not be nearly sufficient to account for the social class gradients observed.

The second observation relied on the concept of social mobility due to ill-health. Thus people who had become ill would, in this explanation, drift down the social class scale. Consequently, there would be a greater proportion of people with disease in the lower social classes compared with the higher, and death rates would simply reflect this difference. Social class, *itself*, however, would not play a *causal* role in the observed inequalities. This possibility was tentatively rejected by the Black Report as there was insufficient direct evidence for or against. Since then, however, there have been studies such as the LS, and analysis of two cohorts of people who have been followed up since their birth in 1946 and 1958, respectively, which shows that the level of social mobility due to disease is quite insufficient to explain the findings.

The third explanation invokes the different health-rated behaviours of people in different social classes as the explanation for the observed health inequalities. There is no doubt, for instance, that the rates of smoking are higher among men and women in the lower social classes (see Table 3.1) compared with the higher.

Also there are higher rates of taking exercise in higher compared with lower social classes. Similarly, more men and women in the higher classes regularly eat fresh fruit and vegetables. Consequently, this explanation suggests that it is these and other differences in behaviour and lifestyle that cause the social class inequalities. To address this possibility we need to turn to the findings of two cohort studies that measured health-related

Table 3.1: Cigarette smoking by social class and gender

	Social class			
	I and II (%)	III NM (%)	III M (%)	IV and V (%)
Men				
Less than 10/day	6	6	10	12
10, less than 20/day	9	13	12	14
20 or more per day	7	9	15	12
Ex-regular smokers	33	25	27	23
Never or only occasionally smoked cigarettes	44	46	36	39
Women				
Less than 10/day	7	8	10	11
10, less than 20/day	9	11	12	14
20 or more per day	6	7	15	11
Ex-regular smokers	21	19	20	20
Never or only occasionally smoked cigarettes	57	58	40	46

Source: ONS, Health Education Authority (1996) *Health in England 1995.*

behaviour and social status of individuals and then followed them over a number of years to relate these factors to ill-health and death rates.

The Whitehall study recruited 17 000 civil servants working in various government offices in London and took great care in ascribing each civil servant to one of the four job grades: 'administrative', 'professional/executive', 'clerical' and 'other'. A large number of known risk factors for coronary heart disease (the major cause of death in developed countries), including health-related behaviours such as cigarette smoking and leisure time exercise were measured for each study subject. Causes of death among study subjects were collected as time went on. A gradient for coronary heart disease death was found to reflect the relative status of the four job grades, those in the highest grade (administrative) had only one-quarter of the rate in the lowest (other) grade. Because risk factors had been measured for each study subject it was possible to calculate how much of this four-fold difference was accounted for by differences in behaviours. This showed that at most 40% of the difference in mortality rate was explainable by behavioural differences. Therefore, 60% of this mortality difference *could not* be causally related to the differences in lifestyles.

The second cohort study we need to consider was conducted in Alameda County, California. This study began in 1965 and followed up a random sample of 7000 Alameda County residents. The study is still continuing and has greatly expanded our knowledge of the causes of many diseases. Social status was measured by income and, as would be expected, a gradient in death rates was seen with those with the lowest income experiencing the highest death rates. This gradient remained even after seven health-related factors were taken into account.

It seems, then, that behavioural factors do not fully explain health inequalities based on occupational social class or income. However, we need to be rather cautious in saying this, after all, health-related behaviour or more generally *lifestyle* is observed to be related to social status, whether this is measured as occupational social class, income, education, housing, economic activity or some other measure.

The final explanation for health inequalities was called the materialist/ structuralist explanation. Here it is the level and quality of material resources that an individual has access to that is important. To generalize, those in lower social classes have less income, less education, less control of work and less satisfying work, poorer housing and, more generally, higher levels of stress than those in higher social classes. These factors are interrelated so, for example, less education would lead to less satisfactory work and lower income, which in turn allows less access to good housing. Furthermore, stresses like unemployment are far more likely to affect those in a lower occupational social class.

The authors of the Black Report concluded that for most parts of the life cycle (i.e. childhood, adolescence, adulthood, old age) the materialistic/ structural explanation accounted for the data more successfully than the three other possible explanations. However, Margaret Whitehead and Nicky Hart (who acted as a research assistant to the Black Report authors), preferred not to draw the line between lifestyle/cultural and materialist/ structural explanations as firmly as this. They acknowledged the inter-relatedness of socio-economic position and health-related behaviour, in that changing the first would be likely to change the second.

This, however, should not be interpreted as a down-playing of the socioeconomic determination of health. The final section of this chapter will consider two possible responses to the problems posed by health inequalities.

Two types of intervention strategy

The first of the two strategies may be called the *behavioural modification strategy*. The second we will call the *socio-political strategy*. They are not mutually exclusive; indeed, we believe that to achieve a reduction of death rates, an increase in life expectancy and an increase in quality of life for everyone in a society these two strategies must be integrated. However, there is an asymmetry between these strategies, as it is likely that behavioural modification would become a part of the socio-political strategy but it is by no means equally plausible that the socio-political strategy would follow behavioural modification. Moreover, we believe that though both strategies are open to the charge of utopianism, the behavioural modification strategy is more utopian. This is so because it suffers from the requirement of sustaining itself without economic, social or cultural institutional support. We now outline these strategies separately, but their relationship should be kept in mind.

Behavioural modification strategy

Behavioural modification relies on changing health-related behaviours in the direction of healthy behaviours: quitting smoking, eating less saturated fat and more fresh fruit and vegetables, taking more exercise and so on. The identification of personal behaviour as central to the risks that each of us faces regarding a wide range of diseases has been a triumph for epidemiology this century. For example, the Framingham study was set up in 1949 to enable the identification of the cause or causes of coronary heart disease and stroke. Framingham is a small town in the US state of Massachusetts; its population was known to be well established and therefore less likely to move away compared with the state average. A large (over 70%) number of the town's population agreed to be medically examined and answered a detailed schedule of questions. They were then re-examined every two years and if they became ill their illness was documented. When a person in this cohort study died, the cause of death was carefully investigated and, where possible, a post-mortem was carried out. This study, which continues to this day, has produced a vast amount of information about how specific factors are associated with heart disease or with stroke, and further insights into cancer have also been obtained. The factors identified have been called *risk factors*.

Three risk factors, in particular, have been identified as major causes of coronary heart disease: cigarette smoking, high blood pressure and high blood cholesterol. Each of these risk factors is, in theory, modifiable by changing behaviour. Reducing or, preferably, quitting smoking, eating less dietary salt and eating less saturated fats and more monosaturated fats would reduce risks from smoking, high blood pressure and raised blood cholesterol, respectively.

However it is not as simple as this. The research that has been done on changing behaviours shows that worthwhile levels of change are very hard to achieve and sustain. The Multiple Risk Factor Intervention Trial, often referred to as MR FIT, recruited 361 662 men who, because of behaviour, were in the highest 10% of risk for heart disease. Huge resources were used in this trial to modify smoking, diet and (through use of drugs) high blood pressure. The results, after seven years were, however, very disappointing. There was no significant difference between the experimental group (who had received the special interventions) and the control group (who had not received any special interventions) in deaths or new cases of coronary heart disease.

Later research trials, such as the recent OXCHECK trial and the British Family Heart Study, show that even with high levels of intervention (given by general practice nurses), which are aimed at behaviour modification, the results achieved can be considered marginal for individual participants. The average reduction in risk of coronary death achieved in participants in the Family Heart Study, for instance, was 11%. Assessing this brings us to a general feature of preventive medicine that has been called the *preventive paradox*.

The preventive paradox was clearly described by the late Professor Geoffrey Rose in his book *The Strategy of Preventive Medicine* (1992). The paradox concerns the typically different rewards that a preventive intervention would achieve at an individual and population level. An 11% reduction in the risk of heart disease may be considered too low a reward by an individual for sustaining a healthy diet, stopping smoking and (say) taking more exercise; however, for the population an 11% reduction in death rate from coronary heart disease would achieve at one go more than *one-third* of the 32% reduction in death rate achieved since 1970. At a population health level this would be a massive achievement. This is the paradox.

The lesson of the preventive paradox had been that we should concentrate on the population distribution of risk factors rather than attempt to identify and treat those at high risk. The argument is that: (i) the observation that far more people carry low levels of risk than the few who carry high levels of the risk factor; (ii) therefore lowering the average level of the risk factor would result in a larger decrease in morbidity or mortality compared with focusing only on the few with the highest risk. The implication is that we all should modify our behaviour so that we all contribute to the lowering of the average level of population risk. The population, rather than the individual patient, becomes the focus for preventive interventions.

The difficulties faced by health planners in attempting to engineer such population shifts are enormous. Where are the gears and levers, and what is the mechanism that we need to understand? Though we have a large number of theories we do not sufficiently understand why populations change their habits. Undoubtedly, more widespread understanding of the ill-health caused by behaviour has had a beneficial influence. The massive health education of the population concerning the harmful effects of smoking has contributed to the fall in the population proportion (or prevalence) of smoking, e.g. from 51% of adult males in 1974 to 28% in 1994, and 40% of adult females to 25% over the same period. However, this population decrease conceals the fact that over this period of time women in the lowest 20% of income distribution have not altered their smoking prevalence of around 50%. This is not because these women have not received and understood the health messages about smoking; they are well informed and they still smoke. But to therefore blame them for their own foolishness is to fail to understand the place and meaning of smoking in their lives. Studies of this issue have relied on *qualitative research methods*, where the aim is to understand the situation in depth rather than gather numerical or statistical data. These studies suggest that smoking is understood as a health risk, however, it also provides convenient comfort and is experienced as helpful in reducing anxieties engendered by the hour-to-hour struggles these low income women face in looking after children and just getting by.

Socio-political strategy

Socio-political strategy begins by acknowledging that material resources are causally related to disease risks and the achievement of health. The importance of *relative* rather than *absolute* resources, at least in those societies that have undergone the epidemiological and demographic transitions (see earlier), is strongly suggested by Richard Wilkinson's work on life expectancy and level of income equality. More equality in incomes is related to longer life expectancy. This finding has now been replicated by other authors in a number of different studies using different countries and data-sets. Wilkinson also shows that levels of social problems, such as drug dependence, crime and homicide, what he calls the 'symptoms of disintegration', are also less in more equal societies.

The policies that lead to health are considered to be those that promote full citizenship among all members of a society. More equality in incomes is seen as important primarily because of its social and cultural effects or accompaniments. It is argued that, contrary to conventional wisdom, higher economic growth is a consequence of policies that explicitly attempt to produce more rather than less economic equality. The 'Asian Tiger' economies have been cast in this light by the World Bank. Essentially, more economic equality is seen to lead to an enhanced personal sense of esteem and worth. Moreover, this sense is not achieved by a competitive struggle of 'all against all' but by what is understood to be a shared endeavour.

We have only begun to trace the outlines of the policy responses that would improve our health and well-being but already the political nature of this task should be clear. What is not wanted is some simple-minded conversion of political views merely because there is good evidence that equality brings about improved health and well-being. Not everyone would want to give up a long-cherished view that economic inequality is justified because we are unequal in what we deserve, merit or need. What is sought is that political discourse integrates this knowledge and, that along with the social effects of inequality, the health effects become part of common understanding.

This chapter has covered a large number of issues and has made a preliminary case for a radical rethink of what constitutes health policy. In the next four chapters we will address what are currently seen as the most important elements of existing health policy: medicine, the NHS and the *Health of the Nation* health strategy. By outlining the existing issues we aim to locate them within the public health perspective already traced out in the first three chapters of this book. In particular, the role of public health doctors will be displayed in the central tasks we identify: how to get from existing concerns to an effective practice of public health based upon an expanded notion of health policy and a re-evaluation of the role of clinical medicine.

Case study

The importance of socio-economic conditions on health

There is hardly a public health practitioner today who would deny the strong links between socio-economic conditions and health. The recommendations from the Black Report (1980) have been very frequently cited by many public health and other professionals since its publication. Though neglected for years, recognition of this pioneering work was eventually given (indirectly) by the Department of Health in their document *Variations in Health* (1996). Nevertheless, the key task of public health doctors in the late 1980s and 1990s has been to increase the awareness of decision-makers to these issues and to reallocate resources accordingly. The NHS reforms of the early 1990s (see pp. 9–10) allowed health authorities, at least in theory, more freedom to concentrate on the broader determinants of health than had been the case. So what, in practice, has happened and what, if anything, has been achieved?

A number of health authorities have drawn on the large volume of literature investigating poverty and deprivation and specific health issues. The latter include, for example:

- injuries – a higher rate of unintended (and intentional) injuries in the younger and oldest age groups in deprived areas

- oral health – an increased rate of decayed, missing or filled teeth in areas of high deprivation, particularly if the local water supply is not fluorinated

- infectious diseases – e.g. tuberculosis, hepatitis A in areas where hygiene standards are low and are aggravated by deprivation.

The implications of these, and many other health issues are compounded within specific population groups, for example, one-parent families, the unemployed, older age groups and minority ethnic communities.

To the list of deprivation effects must be added important lifestyle issues such as smoking, excessive drinking of alcohol, lack of exercise, poor diet and usage of drugs. Trends have been worsening in recent years, most particularly with smoking and exercise, despite intensive and coordinated health education campaigns run by many health agencies.

So what can be done? In recognizing the broader determinants of health and the previously limited role of the NHS in acting on these, many health authorities and health agencies have worked collaboratively with other statutory or non-NHS agencies, e.g. local government authorities, the voluntary and private sectors, to tackle many health issues. The formation of these *health alliances* was actively encouraged by the Department of Health as a method for the implementation of the National Health strategy *The Health of the Nation*. Hundreds of such alliances have been formed dealing with issues such as smoke-free environments, activity leisure schemes, actions against drugs, injury control and so on. Many schemes have actively involved public health practitioners who will advise on needs assessment methods, options appraisal and evaluation.

In addition to broad health promotion and educational messages, public health practitioners and health agencies have been working closely with ill people and the public in deprived areas to identify and attempt to meet health needs. A whole range of methodologies has developed in recent years, including use of focus groups and health panels, together with the more traditional patient/public surveys.

The principle of *localizing commissioning*, whereby a range of health and social care needs are identified at a local level (e.g. in a population of 50–150 000) with a range of services being commissioned, has allowed the wide-ranging needs within deprived areas to be more properly identified and served.

A number of forward-thinking health agencies have broadened their alliance partners and are actively collaborating with European partners with whom they can share intelligence and good practice. In the view of the authors, this should be further encouraged.

Notes

For a general introduction to epidemiology see *Epidemiology in Medicine* by Charles Hennekens (London: Little Brown, 1990). Len Doyal and Ian Gough's *A Theory of Human Need* describes a comprehensive approach to defining the objective needs of human beings in order to achieve health and well-being (London: Macmillan, 1991). The Gough and Thomas article described is 'Need satisfaction and welfare outcomes: theory and explanations' (*Social Policy and Administration*. 1994; **28**: 33–56). For the Rockefeller study see *Good Health at Low Cost* (New York: Rockefeller Foundation, 1987), see also *World Development Report 1993: Issues in Health* (Washington DC: World Bank, 1993). Geoffrey Roses' book *The Strategy of Preventive Medicine* presents the arguments for a behavioural modification approach aimed at entire populations (Oxford: OUP, 1992). Richard Wilkinson's work is well described in *Unhealthy Societies: The Afflictions of Inequality* (London: Routledge, 1996). The Black Report and Margaret Whitehead's work is published as *Inequalities in Health: The Black Report and The Health Divide* (Harmondsworth: Penguin Books, revised edn, 1992). The Whitehall study and much else is described in *Health and Social Organisation* edited by David Blane, Eric Brunner and Richard Wilkinson (London: Routledge, 1996). Nicky Hart's analysis of the Black Report is in *The Sociology of Health and Medicine* (Ormskirk: Causeway Press, 1993). The social class and gender distribution of smoking is given in Table 4.5 in *Health in England 1995 – What People Know, What People Think, What People Do*, by Ann Bridgwood, Gill Malbon, Deborah Lader and Jill Matheson (London: ONC/HEA, 1996).

4

What is wrong with medicine?

The popular image of medicine is that it has made great strides in its ability to diagnose and treat disease, and thereby restore health and quality of life to those struck down with ill-health. Patients, for their part, have a duty to seek out and put their trust in the knowledge and skill of highly expert doctors and must, it surely goes without saying, want to get well. Whilst ill, the patient is allowed by all of us to concentrate on getting better, and can therefore temporarily give up other responsibilities, like work or family life. This image of the patient and the patient's rights (e.g. giving up daily responsibilities) and duties (e.g. wanting to get better) forms the *sick role*, an early contribution of *sociology* to understanding medicine. Since this early and very flattering view of medicine, social sciences, particularly sociology, economics and management sciences, have each developed elaborate critiques of medicine. These critiques are by no means complimentary to what might be called 'medicine's self-image' – medicine seen as the only rational and effective response to the ever present danger of disease. Rather, these critiques interpenetrate each other and squarely put medicine in the dock – medicine is seen as full of contradictions and inefficiencies, is self-serving, interested in exercising and retaining power over patients and scarce resources and in all this it covers its tracks by conjuring up a highly technical account of the way disease *must* be understood.

Medicine is clearly under attack from without but in addition it is surely no surprise to suggest that the last two chapters of this book may be read as an attack on medicine from within. This is only partly correct. Whilst public health medicine does articulate a view of health and disease very different from that found in clinical medicine, the critique of medicine it furnishes is more sympathetic to medicine than the outsider critiques. This is not, we believe, due to a professional closing of ranks but rather to the increased understanding of public health physicians of the day-to-day problems, work and motivations of clinicians. Public health physicians have this understanding because they themselves have been trained and have worked as clinicians. A sociological slant on this, if one is needed, may be found in the practice of *ethnomethodology*, a social science that aims to understand the day-to-day world of people in the conduct of their life and work. So, as the next chapter will show, clinical medicine is open to a public health critique but this critique is tempered by a deep understanding of clinical medicine not found (or not used) in the mainstream critiques offered by social sciences.

We begin by outlining a sociological critique of clinical medicine, then turn to an economic and, finally, to a managerial critique. After these we introduce a public health medicine viewpoint that acknowledges the value of some of these social science views but adds to them other views and emphases, constructing a synthesis from the available critiques. In this way we introduce a public health perspective on clinical medicine which is developed in the next chapter.

Sociological diagnoses

There is no single sociological critique of medicine. There are, however, many critiques that display either explicit or implicit evaluations of medicine, 'critique' here being best understood as an academic word for 'criticism'. One very influential and relatively early criticism focuses on medicine as the exemplar of a profession. The central ability of medicine, which distinguishes it as a profession, is its ability to define its own area of work and expertise. Medicine is thus able to designate both what is and is not a disease and the expertise required to treat this disease. The critical part of this viewpoint is that this ability gives doctors a disproportionate amount of power in their day-to-day dealings, especially in relation to patients. This powerful position is seen by many writers as a potential means of controlling social relationships and institutions. Medicine, it should be remembered, was seen by Eliot Friedson, the author of the *Profession of Medicine*, as just a very good example of the process of *professionalization* (defining the problem and its solution). It is professionalization, rather than medicine *qua* medicine, that is being described and criticized in this early work.

Building on this view of medicine as a profession and thus a powerful institution of social control, we can see many subsequent critiques that have identified and elaborated different elements to establish their own brand of distinct criticism. We will briefly describe here two of these later critiques that will serve to illustrate the concerns that sociologists and social critics have seen as important. The first of these is found in the work of the sociologist Nicky Hart, the second in the work of the medically trained social critic Vincente Navarro. These critiques are chosen as two of many available – indeed, as we will see, sociological critique is now deeply self-reflexive, it deconstructs its own foundations as readily as it deconstructs social institutions such as medicine. It would, therefore, be an impossible project to offer a comprehensive or even a representative survey of sociological viewpoints on medicine. We will, however, use a central method of recent sociological practice, *deconstruction*, to examine the nature of the illustrative critiques chosen. Deconstruction here is used as first a description of the assumptions upon which any given critique stands, and second, an analysis of the interests and tendencies that these assumptions serve.

In her book, *The Sociology of Health and Medicine* (1985), Nicky Hart presents an unrelentingly critical account of modern medicine as a noxious social institution. Clinical doctors are identified as the principal actors who maintain and reproduce this powerful but misconceived social phenomenon. The problem is the way disease is construed and the narrowness of the responses that medicine and doctors affirm as legitimate. The world view of medicine, at least the variety of medicine that has dominated practice in developed nations, is the *biomechanical model*. This model is elaborated to distinguish five distinctive features:

1 A predominant concern with cure together with a distinct dualism between mind and body; legitimate disease is organic – located in the body, the influence of mental states is downplayed; even in psychiatry the focus remains organic.

2 An orientation towards cure – through the practice of medical techniques symptoms are worked upon with the aim of getting rid of them.

3 The representation of disease as an alien intruder that is autonomous but is potentially manageable. This representation contrasts with that which sees disease as a product of the person/environment relationship.

4 The view that it is the individual that is the site of disease and the only appropriate level for medical practice.

5 The view that the hospital, clinic or consulting room, i.e. a medical environment, are the only appropriate locations for treatment, rather than the locations where symptoms arise.

The role of a *sociology of health* is given as the identification of the real reasons for the improvement of health; the task for a *sociology of medicine* is the explanation of how medicine succeeded in '"pulling the wool over everybody's eyes", including their own by all accounts' in convincing people that medicine should have a monopoly of health care in advanced societies.

The explanation of improved health offered by Hart begins, as we have done, with the work of Thomas McKeown and, as we have also done, proceeds to elaborate upon the epidemiological implications of inequalities in health and disease. The explanation of the power of modern medical practice, seen as a social ideology, is traced out using the historical record. Historically, medicine positioned itself to benefit from the advances of scientific enquiry, such as the discovery of bacteria and the founding of bacteriology, and simultaneously worked within the emerging political establishment to accrue to itself professional status.

The picture that emerges from Hart's critique is a world unable to come to terms with the reality of the forces that damage health and create disease. The reasons that explain this view are explicit in the biomechanical model, and we now need to examine these from a public health medicine perspective.

First, the assumption that medicine focuses upon cure rather than care is nowadays much less the reality. It is true that high-tech medicine, acute medicine and, indeed, the popular image of medicine are dominated by the objective of cure, but things have changed, and are changing. Chronic diseases such as heart disease, arthritis, some cancers, many psychiatric diseases, and disabilities due to physical causes or due to learning difficulties, are now the more common conditions in those populations that have undergone both the epidemiological and demographic transitions (see Chapter 3). It is simply in opposition to the facts to believe that these incurable diseases and disorders are not catered for within modern medicine. It is, likewise, a partial view and a gross misunderstanding to believe that medicine does not increasingly give room to the reality of mind–body interactions. Indeed, the increasing importance of these interactions are now seen as unremarkable in the study of allergies, in psychosomatic medicine and in areas of research such as psycho-neuro-endocrinology. We argue later that the medical dominance of 'care services' constitutes an emerging problem. Far from the neglect of 'care' modern medicine has colonized the concept so thoroughly that it has narrowed the social institutions and responses routinely available.

The conception of disease as an alien intruder is similarly old fashioned. It simply does not reflect modern conceptions of causality. For example, genetic diseases, such as haemophilia and cystic fibrosis, do not, by definition, conform to this alienation viewpoint. Auto-immune disease, such as some forms of arthritis, also do not meet this simple conception. The modern view of disease places emphasis on the interaction of factors such as environment, genetic constitution and behaviour. The *germ theory* of disease has been radically modified. We argue later that this change in conception must continue to develop to encompass the interpretation of the facts regarding inequalities in health.

The belief that it is the clinic, conceived as a medically specified location, where medical practice typically occurs (and thus the clinic includes the hospital and the consulting room), is historically correct but history has not stopped. Today, medical practice has escaped the clinic and has indeed become a common encounter within the community. Community care for certain groups, such as the elderly and mentally ill, is only one part of this change. Increasingly the site of medical practice is designed to be within local, often domiciliary settings. This change itself needs to be assessed. It is by no means evident that the spatial expansion of medicine is to be wholly welcomed.

The characteristic features of the biomechanical model are therefore parodies, stop-frames of a dynamic historical process. Medicine and medical practices have changed in the past and continue to change. There is one feature of this model, however, which has not changed – the focus on individual-level explanations of disease and individual treatment – and this is where a public health medicine critique of clinical medicine joins this particular sociological version. We will elaborate on this issue in the concluding part of this chapter; here it should be recognized that this sociological critique is valuable to one very important extent: it refocuses attention on the social and economic causes of disease and health.

The critique of the professionalization of health care (via a sociology of medicine) is much less open to a public health medicine counter critique. This critique identifies clinical medicine as a social ideology. It is, surely, the cultural resonance of the popular view of medicine (depicted in television fiction such as ER, Casualty, Dr Kildare, etc.) which provides the most convincing evidence of the success of this social ideology. This success erects great barriers to what we have previously called a socio-political understanding of health and disease (see Chapter 3). It is at least possible that the historical transformation of the biomechanical model, which we observe, will run up against its limits in the continuance of this social ideology of medicine and the medical profession. This social ideology, it will be recalled, construes medicine and doctors as the only rational responses to disease, disability and illness. *Alternative* (or, less oppositional, *complementary*) type treatments are at best tolerated within mainstream medical practice. Yet the increasing popularity of these alternatives has necessitated a co-optation strategy – seeing alternative treatments as complementary treatments is perhaps the most obvious outcome of this strategy. In summary then, though elements of the biomechanical model are undergoing change there remain two central elements: individual level causation and the social ideology of medicine, which remain largely intact. The socio-political view of health and disease will increasingly run up against these barriers and it is a central task of public health medicine to work for the success of the socio-political viewpoint.

Vincente Navarro, in his book *Medicine under Capitalism* (1976) and in later works, presents an internally coherent critique of modern medicine from a Marxist perspective. The biomechanical model (renamed the *biomedical* model by Navarro), especially its individual focus, is said to serve the capitalist mode of production by placing emphasis on individual biological and behavioural factors as the causes of disease. This is said to divert attention from the wider economic and social environment, which is the true source of, at least, a majority of disease states. This biomedical model is, therefore, a legitimization device for capitalism. Moreover, medicine itself has become an industry and like any industry it encourages consumption by astute marketing. Consumption rather than production becomes the arena for public choice – this again is a masterful diversion because it is the circumstances surrounding production that ought to be examined. The self-interests of doctors are served by capitalist economic and cultural interests, and crucially, vice versa. Any fundamental change in the cultural understanding of medicine and medical practice would present a challenge to capitalism and it is, consequently, unlikely to happen without a class struggle which transforms understanding.

Whether we can now accept a sociology derived from Marx – especially its unproblematic reliance on substructure (economics) creating superstructure (culture) – is arguable. Moreover, the form of Navarro's argument is functionalist: biomedicine exists and is maintained because it functions to maintain and reproduce capitalism. Functionalism as a means of social analysis had been much criticized because it does not have analytical space for the real-world observation that societies and social institutions change. Social stasis is not the rule, it is the exception, yet a functionalist account of any social form cannot adequately cope with transformation.

Later conceptions of the way societies maintain, reproduce and transform themselves have largely succeeded in solving a central problem with functionalism – the necessity within functionalism of seeing human beings as simple pawns in a game (society) that pushes them around. Human beings, however, have 'agency', a capability of doing something that is not foreseeable, not readable from the structure of the situation a person finds himself of herself within. This freedom of the person allows both the maintenance and reproduction of the culture he or she is born into but, simultaneously, also opens up the possibility that they can transform aspects of this world so that it can and does change.

Though Navarro and Hart both offer stimulating critiques of a form of medicine (biomechanical/biomedicine), both have left little or no room for agency. This limits their claims for an even adequate real world description of medicine and freezes their critical insights in time.

Economic prescriptions

If sociologists have changed from seeing medicine as functional for, at least, industrial societies – in, for example, the *sick role* described by the sociologist Talcott Parsons – to seeing medicine as dysfunctional for individual emancipation (e.g. Hart and Navarro), a similar change can be discerned in the writings of economists.

Those economists who interest themselves in health and health care systems are a fairly recent breed and they have, unsurprisingly, called themselves health economists. The UK had the distinction of being among the pre-eminent countries of the world for its production of health economists and the level of their academic output. Being a relatively young subdiscipline, health economists have differing views on many issues, e.g. the nature of the agency relationship (whereby doctors act as informed consumers on behalf of patients), the equity objective of health systems, the existence of supplier-induced demand, the effectiveness of clinical budgeting and (in a list sufficient for present purposes) the ability to measure quality of life between individuals.

Health economists have diagnosed that the heart of the problem in the NHS is the phenomenon of *inefficiency*. The definition of inefficiency clearly relies upon a definition of efficiency and it is therefore necessary to give this definition before we go any further. It turns out that there are two types of efficiency: *allocative* and *operational*. Allocative efficiency occurs when the distribution of scarce resource is that which maximizes the valued output from those resources. Operational efficiency (also known as X or technical efficiency) occurs when for a given amount of resources output is maximized or, for a given amount of output, the resources required are minimized. In health terms, allocative efficiency questions might be as follows:

Q1 How much money should we spend on housing, education, social services, and the NHS to get the maximum return in terms of good health status?

Q2 Where should we put this extra £1 billion (housing, education, social services, NHS) in order to get the maximum increase in good health status?

Operational efficiency would be at issue in these two questions.

Q3 What types of treatment and how much of it (e.g. drugs, physiotherapy, psychotherapy) should we spend money on to get the maximum return, in terms of improved health status, in this case of rheumatoid arthritis?

Q4 Given the required output (say 100 persons living a total of 100 years after having a heart attack) what is the minimum amount of money we need to spend, and what should we spend it on?

The UK health economists' basic charge against medicine is that these questions are seldom, if ever, asked by doctors or managers within the NHS, and are almost never answered in the practice of medicine. Consequently, there is inefficiency – resources put into the system (inputs) do not produce as many valued outcomes (outputs) as they ought to have produced if the resources were used efficiently.

The reason for this inefficiency is that economic actors, such as doctors, do not (even when this is possible) act as *utility maximizers*. Utility is a concept derived from the philosophy of utilitarianism, which originated in the eighteenth and nineteenth centuries. Utility is said to represent all that is valued and preferred by an individual and, in consequence, anything that increases/decreases utility, increases/decreases human individual well-being or welfare. Moreover, an originator of utilitarianism, John Stuart Mill, saw it as evident that an increase in anyone's utility is as good as an increase in your own. The aim of any system is therefore to produce *the greatest pleasure (utility) among the greatest number*, pleasure being one of the many synonyms for utility.

The description of utilitarianism given is known as 'standard utilitarianism', other versions are also on offer. The process (i.e. means to ends) has also been thought to possess utility but in the standard version means (or processes) are not given a utility value. The creation of 'process utilitarianism' mends this perceived deficiency. Similarly, because it is quite possible (even probable) that the total sum of utility within any population can be maximized by the majority of people living in utter luxury and subjecting a minority to slavehood, this and other scenarios is seen as morally repugnant. To cope with this 'rule utilitarianism' was constructed – only some means are available to maximize utility, other means (those that are repugnant) are ruled out. There are great difficulties in sustaining any modified version of utilitarianism. For example, rule utilitarianism cannot adequately be founded on the long-run pay-offs from its permitted rules. We will therefore confine our critique to the standard version.

The thing that gives economics, including health economics, its point is the fact that resources of all kinds (e.g. labour, land, money, entrepreneurialism, new ideas, raw materials) are finite. If we do one thing we cannot use those same resources to do another thing. Because resources are limited, or scarce, we are making economic decisions all the time, simply by choosing to do one thing rather than another. If we believe it to be rational for us to get the most out of our use of resources then we are acting irrationally when we use resources inefficiently. The task of health economics is, then, to offer economic actors in the NHS ways of becoming rational and, hence, efficient.

These remarks seem incontestable – we do, surely, all wish to maximize utility by being efficient – it is the only rational thing to do. But the problem with health economics is in its detail and in its indeterminacy. Let's take the latter problem first. The rational economic actor is, in principle, able to calculate which choice to make among a number of alternative courses of action in order to maximize his or her utility. Now this requires information – regarding the amounts of utility available for each of the alternatives and, say, the timing of the available utilities (utility may come immediately for choice A, but be delayed for a month in choice B and so on). Moreover, we need in this situation to be certain that by choosing A (say) we will certainly receive the utility and the temporal pattern associated with A. Quite simply this is impossible (even in principle). We cannot be certain that the world will deliver the quantity and pattern of utility of A; the best we can do is have an expectation, a probability (between 0 for no chance and 1 for certainty) that this utility and its temporal pattern will be forthcoming. Now when we choose, instead of certainty, we accept a risk of delivery (or, –1 risk of delivery, as the risk of non-delivery), but now we each have our own propensity regarding the level of risk we would accept in any given situation. Moreover, it appears that this level of risk acceptance is not independent of the way it is elicited from us. The level of risk acceptance also appears to be influenced by our personal characteristics, for example by age, gender, social class and our state of health. Even more of a problem appears if we value A over B and B over C, we do not consistently value A over C. What this all means is that we cannot measure utility consistently within and between individuals. Welfare economics has long accepted that it is not possible to measure utility between persons but empirical work suggests that this is not even possible for an individual either. This is the problem of indeterminacy.

Health economists describe a number of techniques that, it is claimed, are useful in providing a framework to enable doctors or others to choose the most efficient use of resources among alternatives. These techniques include cost-benefit analysis (CBA), cost-effectiveness analysis (CEA) and cost-utility analysis (CUA). Let us take cost-effectiveness analysis (CEA) and look at its details. CEA is generally believed to be the least contentious technique, so, if we find unbridgeable problems with it, we can be fairly sure that the other techniques will also unravel under a detailed analysis.

The essential first step in CEA is the identification of at least two courses of action (e.g. treatments or treatment regimens) that will produce the same valued outcome. This outcome does not have to be valued in monetary terms, indeed a great attraction of the CEA is the side-stepping of this issue. Rather, the outcome is typically measured in *natural units*, so, for example, the outcome of blood pressure lowering drugs may be measured in terms of millimetres (mmHg) on a sphygmomanometer (blood pressure reader), treatments designed to improve functional abilities like walking could be measured in terms of distance walked in a given time and so on. The procedure for CEA is then very simple in principle: measure costs of the course of action, measure its benefits (outcomes) in terms of natural units and calculate a benefit–cost ratio for each course of action. The more efficient use of resources is then given by the course of action which has the highest benefit–cost ratio. Simple isn't it?

The problem is this – it is just too simple to be useful. Let's start with the outcome (output/benefit) side. What is the outcome that we should measure? It is not obvious even in drug CEAs what we should measure. The two or more blood pressure drugs may lower blood pressure to similar extents but what about their different profile of side-effects, do we simply ignore them so we can pursue our CEA? Likewise the differing physiotherapies may allow the same walking speeds to be attained but what if one regimen seems to be less painful – do we take this into account? It certainly seems reasonable that we should. But if we do then how do we combine the original outcomes (natural units) with these new outcomes (less pain)? At some point we need to value these outcomes, at least if they occur in the more costly treatment (if the more costly treatment also produced less valued subsidiary outcomes we do not have a problem). We need to add benefits for each course of action, thus we have not side-stepped the valuation issue. We also need, in the end, to choose between benefits and costs. Furthermore, whose benefits are we measuring? – the clinicians, the researchers or the one always used in this disease in the past? It is seldom the patients' chosen outcomes that are measured. This is because patients have very rarely been asked by researchers the simple question, 'What do you want from this treatment?' Patient-chosen (also called patient-centred) outcomes present a lethal blow to CEA and indeed CBA and CUA too, for they throw us back (if we wish to settle the matter without local research) on the unresolved problems of valuing different outcomes from different people, aggregating these outcomes and using measures of central tendency (means, medians) to represent the preferences of our patient populations. But such aggregate measures do not represent anything or anyone, they are simply mathematical constructions – we are now a million miles away from the simple decision-aiding tool that health economists claim CEA to be.

The strong programme of health economics is the open criticism of doctors and medicine based upon the claimed irrational (inefficient) behaviour of clinicians. The weak programme dissembles this criticism, emphasizing the help that health economics can offer busy doctors, enabling them to get more out of their efforts.

What is at stake in these criticisms of health economics? The answer is quite a lot. It is obvious that resources are scarce and that we certainly do need to consider costs as well as benefits if we are able to get the most out of using scarce resources. But just because these are real problems it does not follow that we have adequate answers to them yet. Certainly the proponents of QALYS (quality adjusted life years), incentive structures for paying doctors, CEA and so on need to acknowledge the primitive state of their discipline. Health economics has real-world shortcomings: measurement inadequacies; a simplistic conception of persons; and, to limit this list, has a misleading disciplinary hype that promises much more than it can deliver. The so-called strong programme of health economics is, thankfully, nowhere near established. The weak programme is admissible but must own up to the vast distance between this discipline's aspirations and its capabilities.

In concluding these criticisms of health economics we will make a final point. Even if doctors were to accept it, it is completely unclear what the proponents of the strong programme want to happen – perhaps the replacement of the doctor by a *rational economic physician*. This new breed would be able to calculate utility functions (probably aided by computer technology), compare utilities with costs and draw the rational conclusions. The NHS would then become a rational organization and public money, at last, would be used properly. Here is not the place to go into detail about the little we know about how people (doctors included) actually make decisions. Suffice it to say that from the point of view of what is known as *normative decision theory* doctors, like others, are hopelessly irrational most of the time.

Doctors do not act so as to maximize expected utility, they often take actions that satisfy some rather than all of their and their patients' values, moreover, they do not usually gather all the necessary information needed to act. In other words, doctors, like all the rest of the human race, are fallible. Here we may simply thank our genes that we are all fallible, to be otherwise would reduce us all to rational robots. Human agency would be gone and we would live in an utterly strange new world. Lest health economists would be prepared to pay these cultural costs we should remember that there is no possibility of calculating utility adequately for collective choices (the aggregation problem) even if we had sufficient information. It turns out that the weak programme, modified to be suitably self-critical, is the only possible project for health economics now and in the future.

Managerial imperatives

Chapter 1 sketched out the rise of managerial activity within the NHS. It will be recalled that the Griffith Inquiry report (1983) recommended that there was a need for a general management function, seeing it as the best way of getting things done in the vast NHS organization. Consensus management, where administrators, clinicians and public health physicians constituted the executive board of hospitals, and decisions were taken in a consensus forming way, was found, it will be recalled, to be inadequate in several ways. It was slow, tended to avoid confronting vested interests and, consequently, did not initiate innovation or respond well to externally changed circumstances. General management, with one person in overall control (district general manager) and with lower level managers responsible for individual hospitals (unit manager), was considered to be the solution to such problems. Furthermore, slowness and stasis in the face of external problems were only some of the problems in the NHS that management academics and practitioners had identified. Other prominent issues were recognition of medical practice variations, inequities in the distribution of doctors, hospitals and GP surgeries, and dominating all else, the pervasive financial difficulties under which the service operated during the 1970s and 1980s. All these, it seemed, called for a firm management response.

The NHS is a vast organization, it represents around 6.6% of gross national product (GNP), amounting to £38 billion in 1996/97, employs close to 1 million people and (in a much-quoted formula) requires around 3% annual increases in real terms financing to cope with improved medical technologies and an ageing UK population. The NHS, however, cannot very easily be seen as a business. We can see this by asking the types of questions of the NHS that any similar sized business should be able to answer. The NHS turnover of £38 billion puts the NHS in the same league as a large multinational corporation, such as ICI (Imperial Chemical Industries). Let's start by asking, what goods or services does the NHS produce? The answers could be 'improved health', 'longer life expectancy', 'improved quality of life' and so on. We have already (Chapters 2 and 3) touched on the determinants of improved health. The NHS, representing medicine, cannot be credited with the largest share of this outcome, at least if we consider longer life as a fair measure. So what does the NHS produce? The answer to this question is unknown but 'reassurance that treatment and care will be available to each of us when we need it' is surely a strong contender. It is important that we continually ask this deceptively simple question about the purpose of the NHS even though the answer if far from clear.

Pursuing this issue of purpose of the NHS the answer we have offered above explicitly suggests that the NHS should strive to be available to everyone on the basis of need, and that equity of access is therefore an objective for the NHS. Equity was a central objective of the National Health Service Act 1948 and certainly Aneurin Bevan, the central political actor in the creation of the NHS, saw equity as the defining characteristic of the service. Achieving equity, however, has proved to be very difficult. For a start we have to ask 'equity of what?' The answer is that we consider equity of access, equity of use and equity of outcome as the three main possibilities. Briefly, equity of access would mean (among other things) that there would be no geographical inequalities in the siting of NHS facilities and personnel; equity of use would mean that each person used NHS facilities to the extent their need required; and equity of outcomes (or health) would mean that each person's health was improved to the same level by using the NHS.

The NHS has not achieved its equity of access or outcome objectives. Equity of use has been achieved in some studies but not in others. We will consider additional evidence on this issue in Chapter 5. For present purposes though we might recall that equity of health is not consistent with the evidence of inequalities in health discussed in the previous chapter. Equity of outcome remains the major unfulfilled management goal.

Managers are, it is generally agreed, required to manage, and the variations in medical practice issue is a useful example of the way doctors pose managers with management problems. It is consistently found that the rates of many medical and surgical procedures vary markedly by geographical location. Prostatectomies, hysterectomies, caesarean sections, tonsillectomies and adenoidectomies, hernia repairs, coronary artery bypasses and many other procedures vary markedly (sometimes 20-fold) in their rates both within countries and between countries. The question is, why? Possible answers are: differences in need; differences in availability of the procedure; differences in demand by patients for the procedure; differences in medical decision-making regarding the procedure, or a combination of these. Clinical freedom is commonly invoked as an explanation of this practice variation.

The management problem is this. If the difference is not due to differences in need then there is, logically, an inefficiency or an inequity, or both, that requires management action to correct it. If, in particular, this difference is due to differences in decision-making ('clinical freedom') then it is more likely that an inefficiency and/or inequity has occurred. The manager, therefore, wants to know the reason for the difference. But how can the manager find this out? Ask the doctors? But it is in the doctor's interest, surely, to say that his or her rate for the procedure is that required by clinical need. This is not to suggest that doctors are lying, simply that to them their practice of medicine is unproblematic, it is experienced as clinically required. Could the manager consult a guideline or clinical protocol? Possibly, but these are typically national or international documents and cannot credibly be applied at a local level. So what about clinical audit? This is conducted by clinicians so the problem of the possible self-serving use of information or a need-based justification of existing information within the domain of clinical freedom again appears.

It becomes even more difficult when medical practitioners disagree with each other over what the indications for a procedure ought to be. They may disagree to the extent that no guidelines or protocols exist at all. How can managers cope with this? Certainly this type of problem is far away from the problems that business people face in running their firms. Business management models based on cost accountancy and authoritarianism are simply not useful in these clinical situations. This has not, however, deterred some management academics from advocating similar methods in an attempt to tackle the monster of clinical freedom.

Let's be clear on this term *clinical freedom*. We will as a first definition, say that it is *the ability of a physician in collaboration with the patient to choose a treatment or course of action that has the maintenance or improvement of the patient's health as the objective*. This definition is certainly one with which physicians would agree, but, as we shall discuss later, this definition leaves out two important but essential issues: the *effectiveness* of the treatment or course of action; and the *cost* of the intervention. Strangely, management academics and practitioners have been particularly slow in adopting these two concepts as the legitimate means of criticizing clinical freedom. Health economists, too, it can be said, were slow in their recognition of effectiveness as a central issue but, of course, were among the first to wield costs as a tool of analysis. What this means is that health economics has, until recently, simply redescribed and emphasized what clinicians were always aware of (health resources have costs), and managers have worried themselves and others in attempting to control clinical freedom (as in the case of practice variations) without being aware of what they really objected against.

The NHS reforms were implemented in 1991 (until 1997) and this change was, like others, claimed to be necessary to improve efficiency. Additionally, the changes in 1991 were also claimed as necessary to increase consumer (patient) choice, and make the NHS more responsive to consumer needs. We will discuss how far the NHS reforms have delivered on these objectives in Chapter 6. For now we can note that the quasi-market introduced supplier competition into the NHS for the first time.

This competition has transformed the potential for managerial control of clinical freedom. Paradoxically, it has also made the organizational partnership of managers and clinicians a central issue – early 'macho' management has not survived in this new formation. The nightmare of some management academics, who prophesied that clinicians would move into management positions, has happened. Clinical directors (doctors who hold a budget and direct a clinical service) have become the rule rather than the exception. But whether this change, and other changes, will address the agenda of policy-makers (efficiency, choice, responsiveness) is far from settled. It is not evident, for instance, that clinician mangers even accept this agenda as legitimate. Or, if they do, that they perceive these problems the way that management academics and non-clinician managers do. It is no exaggeration to claim that even between non-clinician managers, the actual content of these notions (efficiency, choice, responsiveness) also varies. This might be termed NHS management indeterminacy.

Managers are, perhaps, easy targets. Certainly, the popular image of the health service manager has been far from flattering. Moreover, they have been accused by management academics of avoiding what is claimed to be the real issue – clinical freedom – and have instead preoccupied themselves with issues that do not confront doctors. Some management academics, noting this avoidance, have diagnosed the reasons. They have identified the differences in power between doctors and managers, which is compounded with puzzlement and culture as key explanatory concepts. Puzzlement, here, refers to the fact that medical practice is in many areas not reducible to protocol or the following of a guideline. Culture refers to the rather obvious fact that the public regard doctors not managers as the appropriate experts in their health care. This trinity of reasons interpenetrate each other, each gaining strength from the others. This diagnosis of the management problem is, in our opinion, largely correct. It successfully locates the problem for managers in three social science notions. What can or ought to be done about this?

The central management task, it appears, conceived from the managers' perspective, is to wrest control from doctors, so that managerial health goals (efficiency, choice, responsiveness) can be achieved. But from the clinicians' perspective a loss of clinical freedom would reduce professional autonomy, degrade their work and, sooner or later, downgrade their social and economic status. Not surprisingly then, this conception of the problem produces a more or less open conflict between parties.

What is required, we suggest, is a reframing of the situation, so that the legitimate space for clinical freedom is identified by both clinicians and managers. This will require that managers give up as useless any fantasies of control derived from outmoded industrial management doctrine. Without this strategic refocusing, management will continue to be about trivia and clinicians will continue as powerful but less effective and less than fully ethical practitioners. In the next chapter we outline the legitimate uses of clinical freedom, and we will now introduce this discussion.

Public health medicine and clinical medicine

Let's be clear about what has been criticized and why. We are critical of particular authors who advocate sets of reforms based on faulty assumptions, techniques and recommendations (e.g. the strong programme of health economics) and we are critical of misconceptions, inadequately framed questions and impossible prescriptions (e.g. authoritarian management). In the case of Hart and Navarro, it was possible to take their views as reflective of a wide spectrum of sociological critiques of medicine. The strong programme of health economics is supported by many, but not all, leading academics in this field. Certainly we would include Alan Maynard and Alan Williams as supporters, but Gavin Mooney does not seem to qualify as an adherent. He, in fact, seems to view the strong programme as both unattainable and overrated. In management there are a range of viewpoints regarding the legitimacy of medical authority and practice. Some authors have identified power and control as the central problems for managers to tackle. Controlling doctors is their ideal. Though this approach has theoretical coherence it fails to offer practising managers a practical means of working. Moreover, in failing (or refusing) to understand doctors as legitimate agents for patients it oversimplifies the motivations of doctors, seeing them, variously, as pawns or miscreants in a series of economic and political games. This simplification allows policy prescriptions (e.g. structuring incentives) which are bound to fail because the complex understanding of doctors as persons has been caricatured in terms of behaviourist cue–response psychology.

Naming names is not our way of scoring points. Rather it helps to limit our critical project and clarify the proposition that *clinical medicine can and should learn from a critical reading of social science* as it applies to medicine. Here, we have illustrated what such a critical reading might look like. This is, we freely admit, a *sympathetic reading*, a reading that refuses to see clinical medicine as irredeemably wrong, conceptually bankrupt and structurally self-serving. This sympathetic reading is, we believe, long overdue and must continue if medicine is to be informed by social science.

But a sympathetic reading is not, we insist, the same as an *uncritical* reading. There are things wrong with contemporary medicine and attention to these problems would benefit the ethical practice and public value of medicine. In the next chapter we will begin a discussion on three central problems of clinical medicine: the effectiveness of medical treatments; the efficiency of medical practice; and the social ideology of medicine. Together, our comments will continue to elaborate a public health medicine critique of clinical medicine. Whilst many of these arguments apply to medicine as it is practised in any industrialized and Westernized culture, others will apply only to UK medicine. A truly universal critique of medicine (if that is possible) is, fortunately, not our present aim.

Case study

The need to work with clinicians

For years prior to the NHS reforms (1991–97) the explicit involvement of clinicians in decision-making and resource allocation had been, to say the least, minimal or, at best, marginal. The latter is exemplified by the schemes piloted at six national sites including Guy's Hospital, London and Huddersfield. In this scheme resources were allocated to clinical managers, and their decisions regarding the spending of their budgets monitored. These schemes were the forerunners of the *clinical directorates* set up after the introduction of the reforms.

The fast moving changes within the NHS, most particularly in the move towards a primary-care led NHS, and the increasing emphasis on improving clinical effectiveness, and the need to base decision-making on sound evidence have all demonstrated the increasingly important need to not only work with clinicians but many other health professionals. Increasingly, as we have demonstrated in this chapter (and will continue to do so in the next), collaboration with clinicians is needed on a wide range of issues notably from advice to a health authority or NHS trust (most particularly from directors of public health and medical directors as well as general practitioners) to initiatives concerned with clinical audit and the outcomes of health care. The moves within the NHS during the mid-1990s to a primary care focus have led, interestingly, to a renaissance of GP involvement in authority and trust decision-making. The explicit emergence of GP fundholders and a variety of GP commissioning groups in the purchaser–provider system in the NHS also, of course, has highlighted the clear need for working closely in ensuring the best use of resources.

The many different areas in which clinicians were becoming involved within the NHS led to the publication, in 1995, of definitive guidelines by the NHS Executive: *Ensuring the Effective Involvement of Professionals in Health Authority Work* [HS6(96)11]. In this document the areas where the effective involvement of clinicians (and, of course, other health professionals) were stated to be particularly important included:

- strategic development and reshaping of services, including health promotion and disease prevention and potential collaborative service provision by trusts

- developments of primary care services and prescribing practice, and support for and monitoring of these

- health needs assessment, priority settings, commissioning, purchasing and contracting decisions

- initiatives concerned with effectiveness, audit and outcomes of care and securing professional requirements regarding clinical practice through contrast specifications

- education and training of professional staff

- building effective health alliances with other organizations, e.g. local authorities, voluntary organizations, commerce and industry

- involving the community in discussion about health needs and service provision.

Another, more succinct, way of interpreting this guidance is to recognize that clinicians and other health professionals should become involved in all working areas of health authorities.

There is no doubt that since the publication of these guidelines many health authorities have made strenuous efforts, with varying degrees of success, to work with clinicians in these areas. The most productive of these have probably been in developing primary care services and in certain purchasing and contracting decisions. Hospital clinicians have, most notably and successfully collaborated with the NHS management in the field of research and development (R&D) with the result that a national R&D programme has been established.

However, there have been areas where lack of involvement of clinicians or, indeed, conflict with them still exists. These particularly have concerned service provision by trusts and issues around 'priority setting' or (as we shall elaborate in the next chapter) rationing of health care. These areas, of course, are closely allied to the important question of clinician morale. Undoubtedly, the initial style of *macho management* after the publication of the Griffiths report (1985) led to frequent conflicts with doctors. The introduction of the NHS reforms also contributed to this falling out. Moreover, there were strong ideological attempts at that time for de-professionalization. However, the 1990s has seen a maturing of NHS management and recognition of the need for closer work with all professional groups. This is reflected in a slow but gradual improvement in clinician morale. There remain exceptions, of course, particularly among GPs who, whilst welcoming the primary care focus within the NHS, have not, so far, necessarily seen associated resources allocated to this changed priority and do not necessarily possess the management skills to deploy existing resources.

Post reforms, and whatever configuration may result from future reviews, there remains a great potential for effective and productive work with clinicians. In collaboration between health professionals and management there remains a need for mutual respect. The crude critiques of professionalization did not recognize this and have not been influential in practice. Public health physicians will undoubtedly continue to have an important role here, not just for their knowledge and skill in rational health care provision but also their ability to act as consensus formers for medical viewpoints.

Notes

The sociological critique of the biomechanical model of medicine can be found in *The Sociology of Health and Medicine* by Nicky Hart (Ormskirk:

Causeway Books, 1985), Vincente Navarro's major statements on the structural flaws and state uses of biomedicine are in *Medicine under Capitalism* (London: Croom Helm, 1976), and *Class Struggle, the State and Medicine* (London: Martin Robertson, 1976). On ethnomethodology see the original statement of its research project *Studies in Ethnomethodology* by Harold Garfinkel (Englewood Cliffs: Prentice Hall, 1967). For a critique of functionalism and a description of 'Structuration Theory' see Anthony Giddens' *The Constitution of Society* (Cambridge: Polity, 1984). For health economics, see Alan Williams' article, 'Economics of coronary artery bypass grafting' (*BMJ*. 1985; **291**: 326–9); *Competition in Health Care Reforming the NHS* by Culyer A J, Maynard A, and Posnett J (London: Macmillan, 1990); *Economic Appraisal of Health Care* by Drummond M (Oxford: OUP, 1986). For a particularly informed account of the state of health economics and a 'weak programme' approach see Gavin Mooney's *Key Issues in Health Economics* (London: Harvester Wheatsheaf, 1994). A brilliant analysis of health economics' assumptions and its typical practical problems can be found in *Health and Efficiency – A Sociology of Health Economics* by Ashmore M, Mulkay M, Pinch T (Milton Keynes: Open University Press, 1989). For two very different management perspectives see Stephen Harrison, David J Hunter, Gordon Marnoch and Christopher Pollitt's *Just Managing: Power and Culture in the National Health Service* (London: Macmillan, 1992) and, Lynn Ashburner and Louise Fitzgerald in Scarborough H (ed.) *The Management of Expertise* (London: Macmillan Business, 1996).

5

How should medicine develop?

Three issues of medicine are discussed in this chapter: effectiveness, efficiency and social ideology. The practice of public health medicine within medicine confronts these issues as centrally important for improving the contribution of clinical medicine to the public's health. Before we consider each issue in detail some general comments will help to provide a context for our discussion.

In previous chapters we have argued the case that medicine has not been, and is not, the main determinant of health. Furthermore, it has not, in its development within Western industrialized countries, been as concerned about the causes of diseases as it has been about the effects of disease. Pathology (the study of the effects of disease) rather than epidemiology has been the guiding science of Western medicine. Consequently, both preventive medicine and health promotion have not been given the resources and the intellectual status they are due. Unsurprisingly then, public health medicine, which uses epidemiology and social sciences in furthering preventive medicine and health promotion, has not been a high status discipline within medicine.

Epidemiology, though, has a use that, potentially, might prove to be devastating to the self-image and self-esteem of medicine. It will be remembered that one of the uses of epidemiology and tasks for public health medicine is the evaluation of clinical treatments. Such an evaluation asks the question, 'Does this treatment (therapy, course of action) work?' It is potentially a devastating question for medicine because if the answer that emerges is 'no', then what legitimacy does the treatment base itself upon? If the claims of a medical treatment to be effective are not supported by a scientific inquiry then, surely, that part of medical practice is of no greater worth than a nostrum sold by a quack.

The injury to medicine's self-image and the public's decreasing respect are two likely consequences of the identification of ineffective practices, but there is another, even worse possible consequence – what if instead of doing no good the treatment does harm? The public's repulsion and rejection of medicine would surely follow such revelations. So the stakes are high in this area. Evaluation of medical treatments is both a scientific and a moral issue. Public health medicine thus poses evaluation questions that go to the heart of medicine's self-image and, potentially, is a challenge to the power of medicine.

Scarce resources are a fact of life. *Opportunity cost* (which means that the real cost of doing something is not doing the next most preferred thing) is a logical concept, and efficiency, whether allocative or operational, is something we all would prefer if we could achieve it without diminishing our experience of utility. These statements are all derived from economic theory and are rather unsurprising. The difficulty, as we discussed in the previous chapter, is applying these pristine concepts to real life, or at least real life medical practice. The problem for economics, and health economics in particular, is that it has not developed a sufficiently adequate conceptual base. In particular, it typically redescribes real problems as a simplified and over-abstracted economic problem. It is this translation that at once makes a real life problem resolvable and, just as likely, makes the resulting answer either unacceptable, utopian, unimplementable or some combination of these.

Nevertheless, by expanding health economics to include other perspectives such as ethical considerations, political interests and epidemiological insights, a real life 'good-enough' method emerges for efficient resource planning and use. One technique that incorporates these insights is marginal programme budgeting (MPB), which we will describe in the second part of this chapter.

Finally, the current social and cultural standing of medicine presents a problem for the social understanding required to bring about a really effective health policy. The socio-political model of health, described in Chapters 3 and 4, does not privilege medicine. Far from locating the causes of disease as alien and independent from the economic and social position of the person, the socio-political model understands economic and social positions and the mechanisms that generate these as centrally important in establishing an individual's risk of disease. By not acknowledging this new paradigm, clinical medicine *de facto* avoids engaging in debate about how our society should work. Public health medicine has a role in trying to unlock this impasse and we will outline some of the first steps towards this in the final part of this chapter.

Archie Cochrane's random reflections

In the Rock Carling lecture of 1971 the Director of the Medical Research Council's Epidemiology Unit, Cardiff, A L ('Archie') Cochrane, identified three fundamental problems of medical practice. Entitled *Effectiveness and Efficiency – Random Reflections on Health Services*, the problems were: (1) the measurement of effectiveness of medical treatment; (ii) ensuring the 'optimum use of personnel and materials in the use of these effective treatments' (this is what Cochrane called 'efficiency'); and (iii) ensuring equality in the NHS.

In setting out effectiveness and efficiency as two useful indices, Cochrane became aware that they were applicable to only part of the NHS. He says:

> I see the NHS, rather crudely, as supplying on the one hand therapy and on the other board and lodging and tender, loving, care. My two indices are very relevant to the former, but only to a limited extent to the latter. I needed another index with which to compare the two branches of the NHS and add a little humanity to my approach. Returning to my early enthusiasm for the idea of an NHS, I soon discovered what I wanted: equality.

Equipped with these three indices, effectiveness, efficiency and equality, Cochrane was able to mount a very influential critique of medicine from within medicine. The overall problem was stated in a rather bizarre anecdote:

> I once asked a worker at a crematorium who had a curiously contented look on his face, what he found so satisfying about his work. He replied that what fascinated him was the way in which so much went in and so little came out. I thought of advising him to get a job in the NHS, it might have increased his job satisfaction ...

The NHS illustrates this input/output discrepancy because within it not only were effective treatments being applied inefficiently but there was also a considerable use of ineffective therapies. This led, in Cochrane's phrase 'to the nicest possible type of inflation'. By this he meant that inefficiency (input inflation) had become a feature of what was still, in its aims and values, a great and worthwhile institution – the NHS. Nevertheless, this was still inflation, characterized by the evidence of more and more resource inputs but static outputs. The solution, he suggested, was the scientific evaluation of therapies, specifically by means of the increased and eventually routine use of the randomized controlled trial (RCT).

The RCT is a technique which enables the specific effects of an intervention (treatment, therapy, etc.) to be identified and measured. The essential design element is *randomization* of the study subjects (patients) into the *experimental* group and *control* group. Consequently, in a typical RCT a patient has a 50:50 chance of being allocated to the intervention (experimental) group or to a control condition. The control condition may be either a placebo (a non-active intervention) or an already existing treatment. For example, in an RCT of a new treatment for migraine the control condition could be either a placebo (e.g. vitamin C) or an established treatment (e.g. paracetamol).

Cochrane is clear that in establishing whether an intervention is effective the only acceptable evidence is the RCT. Moreover, he was clear that RCTs alone were not enough. Treatments should also be costed:

> The main job of medical administrators is to make choices between alternatives. To enable them to make the correct choices they must have accurate comparable data about the benefit and cost of the alternatives. These can really only be obtained by an adequately costed RCT.

The quest for *cost containment* in health services has taken many forms – peer reviews, managed care plans, efficiency drives – none of these, however, has more basis in the scientific culture of medicine than the search for effectiveness. This is closely connected to efficiency because before any other savings are sought and before explicit rationing is introduced it is both an ethical and a professional imperative that ineffective therapies are identified and discontinued. Yet, as Cochrane stated, therapies that have been used for years gain a certain invulnerability. It is seen as unethical to stop them. This is particularly the case in fatal diseases – at least medicine, and doctors, are seen to be doing something, even if that something does not improve the outcome.

New therapies, however, have no ethical or sentimental defences. They must be evaluated by the best scientific means possible. Often, but not always, this requires an RCT. Nowadays this understanding of the need to scientifically evaluate new, and, where possible, existing therapies (or to use a more inclusive word *technologies*) is widespread among health policy advisors and public health practitioners.

It is gaining ground, too, among clinicians. Indeed a group of clinicians (who had also trained in epidemiology and statistics), have worked to create a culture of *evidence-based medicine* (EBM). The founding book on EBM was written by Professor Dave Sackett and his colleagues from McMasters University, Canada, and is entitled *Clinical Epidemiology – A Basic Science for Clinical Medicine* (1992). EBM is based on the axiomatic principle that medical practice should be founded upon adequate and appropriate evidence – this is, of course, Archie Cochrane's modest proposal.

Cochrane's influence on the EBM movement is commemorated in the name given to a current international project that aims to collect RCT evidence on the treatment of each and every disease. The vision of this *Cochrane Collaboration* is that eventually there will be scientific evidence for each and every activity that a clinician engages in. This Collaboration has established the *Cochrane Library*, a series of computer databases of RCTs and meta-analyses of RCTs. Meta-analysis is a statistical method for combining the results of appropriately similar RCTs so that their validity is increased. The Cochrane Library is a long-term project but already there are areas of medical practice, for example in antenatal care, childbirth and neonatal care, which have been systematically evaluated for effectiveness.

Certainly the establishment of the Cochrane Library is a great step towards a rational practice of medicine but there remain problems. For instance, there may not be any RCTs, or RCTs that do exist concerning a disease may not be of adequate scientific quality. Again, RCTs can only answer the questions they were designed to ask, in particular, if an outcome was not specified as the outcome to be measured in an RCT then no evidence about the outcome is available. Moreover, the indications for applying the treatments found to be effective in an RCT (or meta-analysis) are not straightforward. Populations differ in all sorts of ways. The RCTs may have excluded certain groups – so how can you be sure that their results apply to your patient?

It is because of these problems that the dream of the rational economic physician (see Chapter 4) is as far off as ever. The practice of EBM requires two elements: (i) knowledge of the relevant evidence; and (ii) appropriate application of that evidence to the clinical situation. It is the second of these unavoidable steps that requires clinical experience. So, though the Cochrane Library will undoubtedly increase rationality within medicine it does not eradicate the need for experience; indeed it probably makes it more, rather than less, central.

Rationing medicine – technique, ethics, politics?

Health care systems all over the industrialized world suffer from inflation; the NHS is no exception. What is exceptional is that whereas the UK spends around 6.6% of GNP on the NHS, much higher expenditures are the rule in other countries, e.g. 8% in Germany, 8.6% in The Netherlands, and over 12% in the USA and rising. These higher expenditures are not systematically linked to higher performance, measured in terms of health indicators such as mortality and life expectancy. The principal reason for the relatively low UK spending on health is that the NHS has a general practice service that is able to act as a gatekeeper to high cost specialist/hospital care.

An assumption central to explaining health care inflation under current circumstances is that demand is unsatisfied and that 'new products', such as new medical technologies, have an eager public willing and ready to consume them. Certainly this may explain inflation in part, however, the health care 'market' has its own characteristics that complicate this free-market picture.

The first way that health care differs from other products is that there are large differences in knowledge between buyer (patient/public) and seller (doctor/professional). Doctors have had a long training and come to understand the pathology of disease. Moreover, the traditions of medical practice – the one-to-one relationship developed in the medical consultation – is asymmetrical, the doctor has more power because he or she has more knowledge. Even though many patient movements have struggled successfully for greater equality and have shifted this balance, the asymmetry is still a reality. This knowledge gap is, then, the principal reason that health care cannot be equated with marketable goods.

Moreover, in health care the supplier has the opportunity of selling lemons. There may be no market for lemons, but if the supplier has power to redefine lemons as oranges (and there is a market for oranges) then lemons masquerading as oranges are bought. Lemons in this context are ineffective therapies (whether harmful or not). Hence the State's interest in licensing doctors through a system of education and training which provides practitioners with credentials to practise. Hence, also, the elaborate systems of ethical principles that professions devise and promulgate among their members, at once demonstrating self-regulation and assuaging public fears.

However, it may surprise some readers to learn that up until the last 20 years the idea of clinical freedom was not tempered by the absolute ethical principle that the offered therapy should work. Consequently, there has been enough freedom for widely different clinical decision-making regarding any given disease – this results in medical practice variations – and widely different costs incurred by patient, insurance company or State system.

It follows from this that it may well be that the demand for health care is not infinitely expandable or, even with current resources, unsatisfiable. If consumers (patients) were given sufficient and understandable information regarding the effects – good and bad – of available therapies, then it is, we suggest, likely that Western health care systems would satisfy all of the resulting demand for cure. For in this new system patients would be told that many therapies had no scientific basis – no evaluation based upon the RCT. The bulk of decisions would then be about care rather than cure. This is a necessary transformation for modern medicine.

Cochrane was clear that the NHS produced three types of output or outcome: social outcomes, equality outcomes, and therapeutic outcomes. Until now we have concentrated on therapeutic outcomes, as Cochrane did, but we must remember that this is so because, though difficult, therapeutic outcomes were believed to be easier to measure than the other varieties. This belief is not as easily held today as it was in 1971. It is, at least, as possible (or as difficult) to measure social outcomes, such as those specified by Cochrane: 'freedom from worry about the cost of medical treatment and care', 'increased equality between social classes and between different parts of the country', and 'improved care for those who cannot look after themselves'. At least two of these outcomes rely on subjective responses from those who may experience or have experienced health care. They can be measured by asking the appropriate questions in an appropriate way and there is also every opportunity for these outcomes to be measured in different types of system, thus allowing different systems to be compared with each other on outcomes as well as costs. Even though equality in social class and geographical therapeutic outcomes have not been achieved (see Chapters 3, 4 and 6) they remain coherent objectives for the NHS.

Summarizing the discussion so far, we suggest that information on 'cure' (therapeutic outcome) should be routinely available to every potential consumer of health care. This, we suggest, would be likely to reduce demand for very many types of existing but unproven services. Therapeutic outcome must, however, be discussed alongside the two other kinds – social outcomes and equality outcomes. The pattern of work of the NHS would, we suggest, be radically altered by these discussions between doctors and patients. We will elaborate on this in the final part of this chapter. What we suggest overall is that rationing of medical care is not an inevitable requirement. It depends largely upon the current imbalance between doctors and patients regarding information on outcomes.

Further studies on social outcomes are necessary so that different configurations of care, such as that provided by non-health care workers, relatives, friends and so on, can be compared with more traditional (medical/nursing) patterns. With the exception of mental health services it is by no means obvious that care services should be bounded by any type of medical model once care is conceptually separated from cure. Such a separation may result in less or more costly services, but again it is our view that in total the demand for cure and care services will not outstrip a feasible allocation of resources to the reconfigured NHS.

This is just as well because health economics does not provide any technical fix for the ethical and political issues raised by the interrelated topics of priority setting and rationing of cure and care services. There are hardline health economists who persist in stating and restating the truths of economics. These truths are: that choices must be made if resources are scarce; that efficient resource allocation is ethically superior to inefficient allocation, and, given these truths, that just because it is possible to intervene effectively it does not mean that we ought to intervene. It may be inefficient and unethical to do so.

These truths, however, do not include the third central concept of welfare economics (a larger domain which includes health economics), equity. This is so because considerations of equity complicate the pristine mathematical doctrines of the market. Even so, the market remains the central construction of classical and neo-classical economics. Simply put, given a perfect market, the outcome of the activities of buyers and sellers will result in a *pareto optimum*. A pareto optimum occurs when it is not possible to increase the utility of one person without decreasing the utility of one or more others. The problem, however, is that pareto optimality does not rely on any consideration of equity, i.e. the justice or fairness of the resulting (pareto optimum) distribution is not considered. A pareto optimum, for example, could theoretically exist if one person had all the resources and wanted them all; taking anything away from this person would decrease his or her utility and thus the morally necessary redistribution would not itself be a pareto optimum.

Introducing distributional fairness into economics puts paid to the mathematical certainties of market clearing processes. It re-introduces politics and ethics into the problem of allocation and the results are, it seems, just too messy for hard-liners. But by re-introducing (or better, recognizing) politics and ethics in relation to rationing decisions, we are only recognizing the reality of the problem, not solving it. Even if, as we asserted earlier, a focus on doctor–patient information for cure (therapeutic outcomes) would result in the reconfigured NHS being able to meet informed demands for cure and care, there is still a problem of fairness. This problem arises because, as we saw in previous chapters, health, disease risks and ill-health are patterned by social, economic and, indeed, biological (gender, race) variables. Given this distribution, some inequalities (social and economic) could be tackled to level up health status. Now the reconfigured NHS would be able to produce a pareto optimum, but only because a socio-political health policy had already produced a 'level playing field'.

We can usefully extend the discussion in this section by briefly describing a real-world rationing technique that gives space for political/ethical considerations in addition to epidemiological evidence of effectiveness. This marginal programme budgeting technique is applicable at a policy level, not at a practice level. This is both an advantage (it can set out a policy backed by a clear and legitimate account of its derivation; this policy provides the limits for individual practitioner action and, thus, may facilitate its implementation) and a disadvantage (the real action is at practice level; the patient and doctor may think that they are rendered powerless – and they may be right to think this). However, despite the disadvantages of this technique for practitioners and patients it does at least provide a narrative account of the reasoning through which it appeared.

This reasoning forms the basis of our recommendations concerning the doctor–patient discussions in a reconfigured health system. Such discussions can equip patients to understand (though not necessarily agree with) the information on effectiveness and the values that have meant that he or she will not receive what they initially thought was available. As we have discussed, patients may well believe that a therapy will produce an outcome that they desire, but in the majority of cases (and despite the Cochrane Library) this is not correct. By making the discussion of this a part of the consultation the patient is empowered by this knowledge even though he or she may be saddened by their situation. Care, rather than cure, is of course always required in such situations, but care, as we have already suggested, may in many cases be better given outside a formal setting and by people who are not professional health workers.

Marginal programme budgeting (also known by other names, such as programme budgeting and marginal analysis) essentially provides a workable framework for priority setting (and thus rationing). The first step is to decide on what constitutes a 'programme'. This might be, for instance, all treatments and services for people with arthritis, or all treatments and services for cancer, skin disease, heart disease, and so on. Once a programme is specified, the next step is to divide it up into 'sub-programmes'. For instance, the 'Cancer Programme' could be divided up into preventive measures (breast, cervical cancer screening, prostate cancer specific antigen screening), curative measures (e.g. radiotherapy, chemotherapy, surgery) and care services (e.g. psychological support, hospices). The work of a health authority can thus be divided into separate programmes and each programme subdivided. What we then have is a map of activities.

Next we want to have a real-world method of doing marginal analysis. The margin in economics is defined as the costs and benefits that accrue from the production of one further unit of output. A process is efficient when the cost of this marginal production just equals its benefits; any further production would result in more costs than benefits and so would be inefficient. Algebraically it can be shown that with a number of programmes the allocational efficiency becomes optimal when each programme has achieved this marginal cost–benefit equality, i.e. marginal cost = marginal benefits.

But getting the real-world data for marginal analysis is very difficult (see the earlier discussion of cost-effectiveness analysis). So in practice we can set up a panel of judges who can then come up with a 'wish list', which specifies within each programme how they would like to spend an extra (say) £10 000 (the 'incremental wish list'), and also ask them to come up with a wish list which specifies what they would cut if they had £10 000 less to spend ('decremental wish list'). Obviously what has to happen is that for each item specified in each wish list, the costs of doing it (costs incurred) or not doing it (costs saved) are then equated as the benefits of doing it and of not doing it, respectively. The drawing up of these wish lists should be informed by a weighing up of the available evidence on effectiveness together with the explicit use of value judgements regarding equity, merit, avoidance of pain and so on.

We can also ask our panel to judge between programmes, e.g. should we take £10 000 away from cancer and give it to mental illness? It will be apparent that values play a large part in these procedures. As stated, therefore, these value judgements should be informed. This means that the panel must have all the available evidence regarding each sub-programme item. Is it effective, partially effective or ineffective? How much does it cost in money terms? How lethal is the underlying condition without treatment and with treatment? Each of these pieces of information may be only partially available or completely unavailable, so judgement (best guesses) will be required. Some proponents of marginal programme budgeting suggest that equity and other ethical considerations must be applied after the wish list stage, but this is not necessary. Equity may be valued alongside other values and can be applied consciously by the panel of judges in composing their wish lists. To apply equity afterwards is to privilege the wish list procedures and make them appear more objective than they could possibly be in practice.

From these procedures, value-laden priorities will emerge. These priorities form the actions of health authorities when they have extra income, or (more likely) when they have less income. These priorities have been arrived at through a systematic process, the values informing the choices have been identified and weighed against each other (thus conforming to the ethicist's dictum 'only a value can trump a value'), and these considerations together form the legitimizing story. This story is available to justify the choices. Those who disagree with the choices made must argue their case in a similar manner – this is, of course, what constitutes politics. Because each judge's values cannot be presumed to be the same, or even similar, there is a need for their consensus choices to be compatible with an ethical basis for choice. For institutions (and for people), the first ethical imperative is to be just.

What, then, is justice? The work of John Rawls and Brian Barry has clarified this question and has provided a persuasive answer. Rawls, in his book *A Theory of Justice* (1971), carefully constructs an elaborate argument that identifies justice with fairness. In his version of a social contract theory he asks us to imagine ourselves into what he calls an 'original position' where our task is to come up with the principles of a fair society. However, we are in this original position without any knowledge of our own identities, our own skills or defects. This deficit in our self-knowledge is due to the fact that we are under 'a veil of ignorance'. The reason for this veil of ignorance is fairly obvious – we do not know how things have turned out for ourselves and we thus cannot be under any incentives to act in self-interest in the sense that we agree to principles only to the extent that we regain our position or do better. Self-interest in itself is not out-lawed in the original position, indeed it is absolutely required for us to be rationally motivated to make any choice whatever. Only a historically strat-egic self-interest (i.e. awareness of one's own outcome) is not permitted. From these conditions emerge the two principles of justice.

The first principle of justice is that each person is provided with equal civil or political rights. The second principle is that every person should have an equal opportunity to advantageous occupational positions and that economic inequalities are to be so arranged that there is no way in which the least advantaged stratum in the society could, as a whole, do any better. The stipulation regarding inequalities is called 'the difference prin-ciple' and it has, not surprisingly perhaps, been the cause of the major crit-ical discussions, both approving and disapproving, that these ideas have received.

What is the relevance of these ideas to health care prioritization? The purpose of Rawls' discussion is, after all, about the organization of a just society, not how the NHS should function. But Rawls' theory is applicable for two reasons. First, health is described by Rawls as a merit good – something we all need to enable us to participate adequately in our society and be fully part of that society. Second, as Brian Barry elaborates in his ex-tended discussion of Rawls and other theorists in *Theories of Justice* (1989), the focus of social justice is the institution. The NHS is clearly the desig-nated institution for UK health care and thereby qualifies on both grounds for our application of Rawls' framework.

The socio-political health policy, primarily designed to tackle inequality, requires an ethical underpinning, and as we will argue in the penultimate chapter of this book, Rawls can be called into service for this. For present purposes, however, we will narrow the focus to the NHS as it is and work out the implication of fairness for the current NHS. The reality of the cur-rent NHS is that it is an under-funded organization that must prioritize (ration) its services in the face of current demands. The NHS is not (yet) our reconfigured NHS – adequate because patients are empowered with information on outcomes. What would a Rawlsian prioritization policy be like if applied to the NHS of today?

First, it would operate on the basis of needs rather than demands. It would seek to empower all patients but would also attempt to make itself more accessible to those who were socially and economically disadvantaged. Services that were effective would be targeted and marketed at those who were socially and economically disadvantaged. Equality of access, use and outcome, based on need, would be the central policy objective of health services, and health services would be at the forefront of the movement which advocated a socio-political approach to equalizing health status. Notice that in this Rawlsian approach pareto optimization is not a requirement (or an outcome) of policy. The difference principle means that inequalities could exist but, in the context of health, the health of the disadvantaged becomes a priority for State action.

This policy mix would be likely to mean that well-off people would go elsewhere for either some or all of their health care. This would be inevitable under the present resource–demand constraints of the NHS. The merit good nature of health would make such behaviour on the part of the well-off just, because this merit good ought not to be denied to any person whatever their economic circumstances. However, in a Rawlsian NHS the demands of those less advantaged would be prioritized because they come from a group that has greater needs, and this would also be just. However, such a two-tier system would only exacerbate the inequalities of society. This paradoxical outcome serves to show that a Rawlsian NHS is not possible in a non-Rawlsian society. It appears that justice in health care under foreseeable conditions of moderate scarcity is not possible without two changes. First, that the NHS is reconfigured so that all patients are empowered, and second, that Rawlsian justice is extended to all other institutions which impact on health. Actions that would bring about a more equal society would therefore further the socio-political model for health.

Given the scope and size of the changes justice would demand one pressing question is, 'Why should we want a just society?' The motivations for justice are discussed in detail by Brian Barry. He follows the arguments from the Sophists of Ancient Greece to modern day moral philosophers, including Rawls. Two motivations capture this long history. First, justice is pursued because, in the short or in the long run its achievement will prove to be advantageous to the individual. This is *justice as self-interest*. The second motivation is that justice is pursued in order that one is able to furnish an account of one's actions without being self-serving. This is *justice as impartiality*.

These motivations for justice appear as opposites, but the first is subsumed in the second. Impartiality is made operative when we ask questions such as, 'What would it be like to be that man (that woman)?', 'What would I want if I were that woman (that man)?' These questions ask us to empathize with other human beings, identify our need with their needs and become aware of their suffering and understand our shared humanity.

Before finishing this section we need to be clear about what the discussion in this chapter, so far, implies regarding the role of clinical medicine in the movement towards improved health for all members of our society. This, in turn, will allow us to set out the outline of a public health view of clinical medicine.

First, following Cochrane, we must hold medicine to its duty to prevent disease, maintain health and improve ill-health caused by disease or disability. This means we must insist that therapies are evaluated for their therapeutic outcomes, their social outcomes and their role in equalizing health status, especially between those of differing social classes. For most therapies, health care technologies and service configurations we should expect adequate evidence of effectiveness on these outcomes; the RCT is therefore the desired research design. RCTs for existing therapies are ethical if there is doubt about their effectiveness. All new therapies must undergo properly designed RCT procedures before they are admitted into routine practice. This is both an ethical and an economic imperative. The outcomes that are chosen as the end-points for RCT measurement should be chosen with care. It is not acceptable for researchers to believe that they know what people want from an intervention – it has been amply demonstrated in empirical studies that patients and doctors differ in their views regarding what is to be considered as a 'good outcome'. Consequently the public must be involved in choosing what outcomes are to be the focus of RCTs and other outcome research.

Second, doctors must share information with patients. Each consultation should be seen as a meeting 'between two experts'. This will, over time, inevitably mean that medicine becomes less powerful in terms of its dominating position in many societies as 'the only way to health'. Increased understanding by the public will lessen their unrealistic expectations about what medicine can achieve. This may cause anxiety because established attitudes will require modification. These shifts in opinion, however, must occur if a realist health policy is ever to be initiated.

Third, a public which understands that clinical medicine has real limits will, over time, restructure its demands on cure services. The NHS would be able to reconfigure itself with, excepting mental health services, a conceptual and organizational separation between cure and care services.

Care services could be provided by many different social groups in many different ways – the need for evaluation of such new services would, of course, remain a requirement for accreditation and State funding. One by-product of this new public understanding would be the exposure of the 'myth of infinite demand', the dogma that sees demands for health care rising inexorably in the face of insufficient resources. Put simply, people who understand that they cannot achieve what they wished for through treatment will not consume, or will not consume as much, as they would if they were ignorant of the reality. Perhaps some doctors will attempt to remedicalize the anxiety that such a reality will engender, but the momentum of the move towards a realist understanding of health is likely to be unstoppable.

Fourth, even though a realist (that is a socio-political) health policy is required to level up health status in our and other societies, its achievement appears some time off. The social ideology of medicine, which we consider below, together with what Le Grand called the 'ideology of inequality' are massive barriers to a realist health policy. In the meantime prioritization and rationing will continue within health care systems such as the NHS. The acknowledgement that these procedures are not amenable to technical fixes (via a mantra-like repetition of the theoretical truths of economics) is a prerequisite for a reasoned and legitimate practice. The political and ethical nature of prioritization and rationing requires that judges are chosen from all types of background; that they become informed about effectiveness, needs, cost and so on; and that their choices are constrained by a reasonable set of ethical principles.

Certainly in terms of allocation under conditions of moderate scarcity (i.e. the current NHS) the two principles of justice which were derived by Rawls seem to be appropriate. In passing it remains an empirical question whether such a targeting of resources towards the disadvantaged would mean that the NHS became less efficient (the dogma of the 'efficiency–equity trade-off'). Indeed, some neo-classical analyses would suggest increased efficiency (due in part to the 'law of diminishing returns') from such a policy. Real-world methods for prioritization and rationing require further research and development, however, the marginal programme budgeting technique seems to be a usable way of proceeding. All such methods require refinement, especially with regard to the composition of the judgement panel.

Medicine as a social ideology

This final section will discuss the assertion that medicine is a social ideology. This proposition has been made by sociologists of medicine and it is an argument partially accepted by us. The topic is important because it provides for the durability and power of modern medicine. A social ideology functions to produce and reproduce a particular set of attitudes and responses among those who accept it as being true. Consequently, a social ideology of medicine is a powerful means through which positive attitudes and responses towards medicine perpetuate themselves. Really successful social ideologies have the character of being taken as 'common sense' – if they are thought about at all. That modern medicine and medical practice is a highly successful social ideology is becoming more and more apparent to those who ask such basic questions as: 'Does medicine improve health?' 'Does medical care extend life?' and 'Is medicine the only legitimate and effective way to health?'.

As we have previously discussed, the answers to these questions support only a very limited role for modern medicine in sustaining and improving health. Yet because of the taken-for-granted nature of the common image (and self-image) of medicine, the image of cumulative progress, therapeutic success and legitimate dominance as 'the only way to health', to raise such basic questions would seem to go against common sense. This is at once a barrier to other conceptions of health (particularly the socio-political nature of causation), and a powerful, if false, argument for the status quo.

The 'establishment' within medicine reinforces the 'common sense' view of medicine. The popular and medical trade media are replete with 'break throughs', 'startling new discoveries' and stories of 'new hope for ———— sufferers' (fill in the blank with a disease of your choice). The pharmaceutical industry is worth billions of pounds and comprises some of the world's largest multi-national corporations. Certainly there are great vested interests in drug development, and in ensuring that these drugs are prescribed and represcribed. The academic institutions participate in the social ideology by their strictures on ways to knowledge and by privileging those types of research effort which reflect what it sees as important. The prestigious research councils announce yet more money available to molecular geneticists, who are asked to use their 'big science' to solve problems like obesity, delinquency, aggression and drug dependence. But why are the most obvious facts regarding health and disease overlooked or marginalized?

These obvious facts have been set out in Chapters 2 and 3. They point to health and disease as socially and economically determined states. The facts point to social and economic causes as generative of behaviours and problems such as smoking, alcohol and drug abuse, depression, anxiety, obesity and so on. The facts point towards a systematic and patterned adverse influence of social and economic disadvantage throughout the lifetime of an individual and its transmission into the next generation. To ask molecular geneticists to explain these facts is to commit a category mistake.

Yet the alternative is probably dreaded by those who stay within the prevailing paradigm of biomedicine. The alternative paradigm is a world where science's claims are put into perspective, where science itself is understood as being a value-laden set of practices whose content and meaning changes as the social context changes. So it is that complex questions of causation are reduced to the types of question that biomedicine can cope with. Rather than attempting to understand the complex social and economic mechanisms which generate the pathways of disease risks, biomedicine simply redescribes the problem and locates it within the body, the cell or the gene. Though social and economic causes of disease must in the end adversely affect the organic structure and function of our bodies, the paradigm of biomedicine concentrates on this final common pathway and thus narrows our ability to prevent the problem arising.

This redescription has, sometimes, paid off. It has, on occasion, identified the final biological pathway of a bio-psycho-social chain of causation, and has thereby been able to block, control or reverse the pathology. But for much of its history, so far, biomedicine has held out extravagant promissory notes of prevention or cure, and has not been able to honour them.

Cancer, for example, still routinely claims the lives of around one-quarter of men and women in countries which have undergone the epidemiological transition. Apart from some childhood cancers (notably acute lymphoblastic leukaemia) and adult cancers (notably testicular cancer and Hodgkin's lymphoma), the prognosis of most cancers has not improved in the last 20 to 30 years. An authoritative estimate of overall survival rate claimed only a 4% improvement during the last 30 years. No great breakthrough in molecular understanding has translated into a new treatment. The modes of treatment for cancer are as they were 30 years ago – burn it, poison it or cut it out. The dream of the human genome project – an international programme that aims to determine the entire genetic sequence of human beings – is fundamentally misguided. Again, what is occurring is a category mistake. Prevention and cure are being looked for in the wrong places.

Things will change. Thomas Kuhn demonstrated that the history of science is replete with changes in the way scientists make sense of their observations; these small changes constitute 'normal science'. The organizing framework (the paradigm) for understanding observations and connecting them up changes much less frequently. But when the paradigm does change it does so relatively swiftly. The new paradigm quickly becomes the taken-for-granted framework for understanding the old and the new scientific data. Kuhn says that with a paradigm change the world has changed.

This is not meant to be a rhetorical claim, it is meant literally. From the perspective of the new understanding (the new paradigm) the way the world *is* is different compared with how it was from within the old paradigm. We suggest that the accumulating evidence for the social and economic determinants of health and disease will in due course effect a paradigm change within the biomedical establishment.

The ideology of biomedicine will not though simply surrender; it needs to be struggled against. Certainly the paradigm of biomedicine will increasingly yield less and less that is useful for improving our health. It will continue to attract those who seek for every problem the 'one true answer' – a biological mechanism, describable in molecular detail – but these molecular details will prove to be indecipherable because they have no context of causation. Knowing the genetic sequence can allow us to synthesize the protein but what do we do then? The relatively new discipline of molecular epidemiology does offer one possible way out of this dead end, but so far it has not been sophisticated enough in the questions it asks.

The predictions we have made about the diminishing returns of a biomedical paradigm may be proved wrong. It may be that for a complex bio-psycho-social problem a biological mechanism can be located and a technological fix (a drug, or surgery, or gene therapy, and so on) can be devised. But we are prepared to bet that this will not occur. We would bet that no gene or polygenetic formation will be found to explain obesity, asthma, schizophrenia, arthritis, cancer of the colon, drug dependence, ischaemic heart disease or any common disease. We do expect that molecular mechanisms will be found and their genetic basis will be uncovered for these diseases. What we don't accept is that these mechanisms will be exploitable in terms of curative therapy or, more certain, prevention. For this, the pathways of causation must be understood, the generative causes within the environment as well as the molecular final common pathways within the body.

What will replace biomedicine? The answer is, of course, unknown but some broad speculations can be attempted. Medical education will change radically; it will attempt to retain the best traditions of medicine with an understanding of the new paradigm. Aetiology – cause of disease and disability – will replace pathology as the central discipline. This will enable clinicians to engage with patients in an exploration of the patient's ecological situation. The social, economic, psychological position of patients will figure as much as the somatic changes that will continue to be identified and labelled as specific disease states. The healing relationship of doctor with patient, which modern high technology medicine has often eclipsed, will be a central achievement of both patient and doctor. In this equal relationship the jargon of science will be demystified, evidence regarding available treatments will be discussed in meaningful and comprehensible ways, and patients will be empowered and supported in their choices.

This new practice of medicine will not medicalize social, economic or political problems. Damp housing, which causes respiratory disease, will be identified as the economic and social cause of disease, the citizen's right to health-promoting housing will be part of the diagnosis, but, of course, it will be a duty of the local politically legitimized authority to effect the transfer or repairs necessary for access to this housing.

Even though the barriers to a realist health policy – which includes a new clinical practice – are large, we have here outlined a possible chain of events. The demise of the biomedical paradigm will inevitably dictate a new clinical practice and the taken-for-granted 'common sense' view of causation of disease will also change. Economic and social generative causes and pathways will be part of the discourse of health and disease. It will be increasingly difficult for political discourse to characterize this knowledge as 'gross meddling' or as promoting 'the nanny State'. All political parties will adjust their policies so that health is safeguarded by each of their policies, whether they be ostensibly about employment, housing, social security or transport.

This chapter has confronted three issues that have the power to transform clinical medicine: effectiveness, efficiency and social ideology. Public health doctors work every day with the first two issues and health promotion is increasingly the area where the social ideology of medicine is raised as a problem. Unlike other critics, public health physicians work routinely with clinicians and they combine a critique of current practice with an understanding of the legitimate claims of medicine. Clinical freedom does need to be transformed; in particular the limits of medicine need to be openly discussed with individual patients and patients must be empowered through this knowledge to choose treatment in partnership with their doctors. However, the central relationship of trust between patient and doctor must be given space in any new way of practice. A transformed paradigm of medicine – from a biomedical to a socio-political perspective – may be some time off, but clinical practice can and should promote and facilitate this change.

Case study

Effectiveness, rationing and setting priorities

Almost since the start of the NHS, there has been an increasing demand for health care. This increase, of course, reflects population growth and changes in the population structure, as well as changes in the underlying prevalence of some diseases. Equally important has been the tremendous growth of new technologies that provide more complex interventions where only simple care was previously available. Many technologies, in particular, provide opportunities to screen and to treat asymptomatic disease.

It is also clear that increasing health care expenditure will not remove the need to make hard choices. The First Report of the Health Committee of the House of Commons on Priority Setting in 1995 established that it was necessary to set priorities in the provision of health care. The Conservative Government of the time accepted this principle and stated in its response to that committee:

> The Government recognises these pressures, not least in its commitment to real term increases in NHS spending. Even so, budgets will always be finite while demand is potentially open ended. There will always be a gap between all we wish to do and all that we can – setting priorities is a fact of life.

However, it also stated:

> The issue of rationing core services does not arise while there is scope for further improvements in effectiveness.

The latter statement is open to some debate, not least as to the definition of *core services*. Our position is that an *informed demand* will be considerably lower than an uniformed demand. In a health system which empowered the public there would be a much stronger imperative that services were effective in patient-chosen terms. However, as a joint document of the Academy of Medical Royal Colleges, the British Medical Association, the National Association of Health Authorities and Trusts and the NHS Executive clearly stated, 'The reality is that an increasing number of interventions, whilst of some proven benefit to the recipients, are very expensive and have a high opportunity cost in terms of the care that has to be foregone elsewhere in the system to provide them'. This fact means that considerations other than effectiveness are likely to be necessary in any foreseeable allocations system.

The authors of the joint report describe choices for health care being made at three levels:

- *macro* decisions are taken by governments about the balance of public spending and the proportion allocated to health;

- *meso* decisions are taken by health authorities, GP fundholders and trusts about the balance of services that will be made available to local people;

- *micro* decisions are taken by individual clinicians in relation to particular patients.

These sets of choices do, however, overlap. For example, individual clinicians cannot choose to offer a service to a patient if macro or meso decisions mean such a service is not available. So, how are health care purchasers, and public health physicians in particular, tackling the effectiveness and rationing debates?

Putting it diplomatically, these debates are providing a considerable challenge to all. As we have seen in this chapter, the rising awareness of the need to demonstrate the effectiveness of health care interventions has arrived not a moment too soon. A great range of initiatives has been set up in recent years within the NHS to tackle this important issue. It is interesting, for example, to document what was recently issued in a 'reference pack' on clinical effectiveness by the NHS Executive:

- details of a second series of *epidemiologically based needs assessments* concerning accidents, cancer, back pain, dermatology, mental health, gynaecology and palliative and terminal care

- details of seven academic centres who have built up a particular expertise in developing evidence-linked clinical guidelines

- details of many national centres offering effectiveness advice

- a list of national confidential enquiries to various aspects of health care

- a list of national advisory committees

- details of professional and NHS Executive contacts

- Effective Health Care Bulletins

- advice on the critical appraisal of reviews

- details of available national clinical guidelines

- details of health technology assessments (that are part of a research programme) which health care purchasers are asked not to purchase in the short term.

Thus, an enormous plethora of advice and information is already available and the literature in this area seems to grow exponentially. Public health doctors are working closely with their clinical colleagues to put this *evidence* into actual clinical care, including varying degrees of multidisciplinary care. The development of clinical audit in primary, secondary and tertiary care bears some testimony to this. However, the growing pace of new technologies and new drugs has added further pressure to the principle of only purchasing interventions where evidence of effectiveness exists. Indeed, many health authorities now use an approach called *conditional purchasing*, whereby agreement is reached in advance of the introduction of any specific intervention what the acceptable evidence for effectiveness should be.

The debate becomes even trickier on the issue of rationing. One of the most publicized cases in recent years was a decision by Cambridge Health Authority not to fund a second bone marrow transplant operation for a 10-year-old girl. Further examples include: whether to fund Interferon-beta for multiple sclerosis patients; infertility treatment for those requesting it; cosmetic surgery for removal of tattoos and varicose vein treatments. In November 1996, the then Secretary of State for Health (Stephen Dorrell) stated that health authorities should not issue blanket bans on any treatment. Some authorities continued to do so but included a clause saying that if there was an overriding clinical need then the procedure could proceed.

Increasingly, and in a way which we support, the debate on rationing is being opened up to a wider audience – both within and, importantly, outside of the NHS. More of the public are becoming involved through media debates or involvement with *citizen juries, focus groups,* or *health panels.* Lessons from other countries that have tackled the issue, e.g. the United States (Oregon), New Zealand, the Netherlands and Sweden, are being widely discussed in the UK. However, as the reference pack authors state: 'It seems unlikely, in view of the demographic and technical pressures and public expectations, that the gap [between resources and demand in the NHS] will narrow significantly. It is therefore inevitable that there will be difficult choices in the provision of health care for the foreseeable future ...'

Our desired reconfigured health system notwithstanding.

Notes

Archie Cochrane's views can be found in his lecture monograph *Effectiveness and Efficiency – Random Reflections on Health Services* (Oxford: Nuffield Provincial Hospital Trust, 1972). The best argument for evidence-based medicine can be found in David L Sackett, R Brian Haynes, Gordon H Guyatt and Peter Tugwell's *Clinical Epidemiology – A Basic Science for Clinical*

Medicine (London: Little, Brown and Company, 2nd edn, 1991). For evidence-based medicine and the need for clinical experience in the interpretation of evidence of effectiveness see, Sackett *et al.* 'Evidence based medicine: What it is and what it isn't (*BMJ* [editorial]. 1996; **312**: 71–2). For the Cochrane Library contact: BMJ Publishing Group, PO Box 295, London WC1H 9TE, for details. The Library Service is supplied on CD ROM format for PCS. For the economic theory of Lemons see Ian McClean's *Public Choice An Introduction* (Oxford: Basil Blackwell, 1990). For a general discussion of Pareto conditions and optimality see John Cullis and Philip Jones' *Public Finance and Public Choice* (London: McGraw Hill 1992). For Marginal Programme Budgeting see 'Public health and economics in tandem' by Madden L, Hussey R, Mooney G and Church E (*Health Policy*. 1995; **33**: 161–8). Note that the authors of this study applied equity considerations after their marginal analysis. We recommend it be integrated with the marginal analysis. An excellent account of Marginal Programme Budgeting is given by David Cohen in 'Marginal analysis in practice: an alternative to need assessment for contracting for health' (*BMJ*. 1994; **309**: 781–4). A brilliant critique of the assumptions of economic analysis is given by Martin Hollis in *Reason in Action – Essays in the Philosophy of Social Science* (Cambridge: Cambridge University Press, 1996). John Rawls' book *A Theory of Justice* (Cambridge, Mass: Harvard University Press, 1971) has been the centre of a critical industry, see for example J H Wellbank, Denis Snook and David T Mason's *John Rawls and His Critics: An Annotated Bibliography* (London: Garland, 1982). For the two traditions of justice see, Brian Barry's *Theories of Justice* (London: Harvester Wheatsheaf, 1989). For a clear statement of medicine as a social ideology see, Nicky Hart's book *The Sociology of Health and Medicine* (Ormskirk: Causeway Press, 1993). For modern views on the status of science see *The Philosophy of Science* (ed. David Papineau) (Oxford: Oxford University Press, 1996). Thomas Kuhn's book *The Structure of Scientific Revolutions* (Chicago: University of Chicago Press, 2nd edn, 1970) remains the best account of how science changes – the paradigm shift. For the claim that no new therapeutic breakthroughs have been derived from molecular biology see 'Evaluating the National Cancer Programme: An Ongoing process'. Presidents' Cancer Panel meeting, September 22, 1993. National Cancer Institute, Bethesda, MD, 1994, see also 'A War Not Won' by Tim Beardsley (*Scientific American*, January 1994). For the cultural impact of genetics see, Dorothy Nelkin and M Susan Lindee's book *The DNA Mystique: The Gene as a Cultural Icon* (New York: WH Freeman, 1995). The Case Study refers to NHS Executive *Priority Setting in the NHS: a discussion document*. *Academy of Medical Royal Colleges, BMA, NAHAT.* (Leeds: HMSO, 1997). The House of Commons Health Committee published *Priority Setting in the*

NHS: purchasing (HC 134-1) (London: HMSO, 1995). See also, Department of Health *Government Response to the First Report of the Health Committee, Session 1994–95. Priority Setting* (Cm 2826) (London: HMSO, 1995). The reference pack was published by NHS Executive *Clinical Effectiveness: reference pack* (Leeds: HMSO, 1996).

6

Is the NHS a success?

What is there left to say about the NHS? This question is aimed at the industry of policy analysts, politicians, economists, sociologists and professional commentators who have intellectually colonized the NHS. No institution is above criticism but the NHS has, since its inception in 1948, received more than its fair share.

So why have a chapter about the NHS, why perpetuate the obsession of the policy analyst? It is because we believe that most policy analysts have missed or have marginalized a number of rather important points in their clamour to describe and theorize about power, change, priorities and the economic trinity of efficiency, effectiveness and equity within the NHS. Our position can be summed up like this. The NHS was founded on sound economic and political principles, and, it turns out, these principles have endured over time. It was (pre-NHS reforms 1991) a relatively efficient organization and it was capable of evolving into a much more effective and efficient one. The period of NHS reforms (1991–97) has not transformed the efficiency of the NHS but it may have allowed an acceleration in considering effectiveness as a central criterion of performance. However, the price paid for this appears to have been an unwelcome cultural transformation within the organization from a broadly collective to an inappropriate individualist culture, and this has had the effect of reducing equity as a goal for the NHS.

What this chapter attempts to do is, first, to take a look at the critiques that have been made of the NHS. This section is not a comprehensive survey, since the focus of the NHS policy industry changes so frequently and so inexorably that this would be a futile and unrewarding task. Instead, through a consideration of an influential commentary on the NHS, we summarize the major trends and tendencies. Second, a defence of the NHS is sketched out. This locates the benefits of the NHS within cultural, social, political and economic fields of discussion. A defence is required to defuse an oversimple public health analysis of the NHS which finds it wanting. Third, the current status of the NHS in the wake of the NHS reforms is outlined and its foreseeable future is sketched out. The chapter concludes with a number of problems and issues that any serious future reform should address.

Whilst our contribution to the understanding of the NHS has a similarity to those produced by the critical industry surrounding it, the selection of issues, their ordering and priority is based upon a public health medicine perspective. This perspective has not so far been allowed sufficient prominence within the critical industry. This, then, is a start.

Problems, problems, problems

The creators of the NHS made what has turned out to be a number of remarkably resilient decisions. The NHS was to be comprehensive, so that it covers all the people of the UK (in contrast to the 1911 National Insurance Act which covered only working men in manual jobs), it was to be free (this has remained substantially so even in the face of prescription and other charges), and it would be funded in the main from general taxation. These three policy decisions can act as fixed points as we navigate the subsequent fate of the NHS.

In tracing the history of the NHS, policy analysts have had a free reign allowing them to isolate one or another series of historical events, create from them a theme and then connect each theme up with social or economic events in the national or international spheres. Thus Rudolf Klein in *The Politics of the NHS* (1983, 2nd edn, 1989) is able to periodicize the history of the NHS in a series of chapters: 'The politics of creation', 'The politics of consolidation', 'The politics of technocratic change' and 'The politics of disillusionment'. The themes Klein constructs are multiple and sometimes ambiguous. Three themes, however, appear to do considerable work in his book running through all the periods considered and ordering what might otherwise be a mass of contingent or loosely associated events. These themes are: (i) the internal/external relationships between the NHS and wider society; (ii) the political nature of the NHS; and (iii) the tension between a rationally planned NHS and a 'muddling through' NHS.

The first theme allows Klein to set the fortunes of the NHS within the wider context of the UK. From wild optimism in 1948 to retrenchment, when the financial costs of the NHS became a political problem during the 1950s. The period 1960–75 is understood by Klein to be one of 'technocratic politics' showing an increasing reliance of society on the ability of experts to identify and solve problems of administration and strategy. This period is seen as rationalism's heyday, and it gave the promise of progressively greater efficiency. Within this period, however, Klein sees the roots of a number of problems that would continue to beset the NHS to the present day: the problem of pay for doctors, nurses and other staff, the perception that the service was 'starved of resources', the search for an 'organizational fix' to deliver greater efficiency and accountability. The NHS in all of this is portrayed as reflecting the wider society; it is a child of its times.

The second theme, the political nature of the NHS, begins with the forging of a broad 'consensus' about the idea of the service and this picture is developed in a series of case studies. These illustrate both the national party politics of the time and the organizational politics of the NHS.

There is ample illustration of the political differences between Labour and Conservative Parties regarding specific issues – pay beds, charges, health insurance subsidies. However, the NHS has historically been an area of political agreement that has transcended fundamental political disagreements. Certainly this cannot be said for other areas of the welfare state, particularly housing, social security and education.

The second edition of Klein's book (1989) includes a chapter on the period 1983–89 and covers the publication of the 1989 White Paper *Working for Patients*, which announced the NHS reforms. What is seen as remarkable is that a highly ideological government, under Mrs (later Baroness) Thatcher remained committed to the founding principles of the NHS. The political costs of a radical rethinking of these founding principles were seemingly too high. The rhetoric of the NHS reforms, though, was radical and so was its central idea, the purchaser–provider split.

In Klein's view, the micropolitics of the NHS is dominated by the interest and calculation of doctors. Klein identifies a central political dilemma – whilst politicians are held accountable for the performance of the NHS, it is doctors who, in the event, control the use of resources. The invention of management systems, such as general management, the NHS planning system and 'accountability reviews' which involve discussion of 'waiting lists' and other 'performance indicators' does not alter this fact.

In his analysis, Klein manages to convey an air of academic detachment and amazes us with his ability to see the connections between apparently disparate issues and events. No doubt his broad conclusions (after the facts) are sensible and his interpretations are coherent but his main attraction of us is to be found in his common sense. The NHS is, and will remain, a political institution, treating it as a dispassionate rational and value-free organization would be simply wrong as well as foolish.

Klein's final theme is most important from both a common sense and a public health perspective. It discusses two central issues: first, the absence of any rational set of planning and evaluation techniques for measuring the success of the NHS; and second, the implications of this absence for the meaning of 'success' when applied to the service. These issues are important to understanding the role of the NHS within a public health agenda and will be discussed in some detail.

The NHS is a complex organization that delivers a heterogeneous mix of outcomes (outputs). This immediately makes any measurement of the input/output relationship a complex task. Despite the attempts by health economists, and others, to convert all of these outputs into a single 'currency' (for example, QALYS – quality adjusted life years), this complexity remains. Quality adjusted life years remain an obsession for some of their originators but are seen as lacking basic credibility in most quarters. Thus we confront a large set of problems. The NHS cannot be judged by its output, the relationship between input and output cannot be specified and we, therefore, have no rigorous methods for judging the performance of the service.

Consequently we have a proliferation of performance indicators that it is hoped might fill some of this information gap – waiting list times, finished consultant episodes (FCEs), turnaround times, length of stay and so on. In the absence of coherent outcome measurements (that is, valid and reliable measures of whether, at least, what the patient wanted from the therapy was achieved and can be attributed to it), any performance indicator can be interpreted as showing either success (e.g. more FCEs, less length of stay) or failure (e.g. more FCEs because of relapse following reduced length of stay). Politicians can thus play statistical games and in this climate others are forced to do likewise.

For example, the Department of Health requires efficiency gains of around 3% per year. This is technical efficiency, i.e. whatever level of output was achieved last year should now be increased by 3% for the same expenditure or the previous level of output achieved for 3% less input. In these circumstances, bureaucratic games are to be expected and are played. Increased throughput, for example, can be achieved by choosing the less complex cases, discharging them early and relying on primary care services for follow-up and so on.

Given this lack of useful information about the outcomes of NHS therapies answering the question 'Has the NHS been a success?' demands a large amount of context setting. Rudolf Klein identifies at least five perspectives for answering this question: the criteria of the founders of the NHS; the achievement of national policy; maintaining and increasing public acceptance and support; administrative efficiency; and increasing public health.

The founders of the NHS set three criteria for the service: (i) it would abolish 'ability to pay' as a barrier to treatment; (ii) it would 'provide the people of Great Britain, no matter where they may be, with the same level of service'; and (iii) the NHS would 'universalize the best (in terms of service)'. These are all equity considerations and the quotations are from Aneurin Bevan.

The NHS can be counted as a great success regarding the first criterion. Ability to pay is not a substantial barrier to treatment. Though it is true that the economic costs of treatment may remain higher for working people in lower social classes (e.g. loss of earnings due to time off work), they may conversely be less for those who are unemployed. Moreover, charges for prescriptions and other (e.g. ophthalmic) services are not levied on certain groups (e.g. pensioners, those on income support) who would find them a barrier to receiving treatment. Overall, equity of economic access has been achieved.

On the second criterion the NHS has performed less well. There remain geographical inequities in the provision of health care facilities. This has prompted Julian Tudor-Hart, a GP and epidemiologist, to come up with 'The Inverse Care Law' – the provision of medical services is inversely associated with the need for services. The Regional Allocation of Resources Working Party (RAWP) was set up in 1975 and devised a formula that included population served and a measure of 'need' (using standardized mortality ratios). This formula was successfully deployed in making regional allocation more equal. However, within regions there remain high levels of geographical inequalities at district levels, for instance the number of GPs per 1000 population shows a striking variation. Moreover, in terms of personnel and facilities there remain substantial regional inequalities.

Furthermore, survey evidence has shown that working class patients receive less time in consultation with their GPs, receive less investigations and less specialist referrals than higher social glass groups. This has been interpreted to show a 'culture gap' between patient and doctor. More importantly there remain systematic social class differences in the mortality rates of patients who receive NHS treatment in a number of diseases – cancer and coronary heart disease are the most prominent examples. Inequities in the quality of treatment have also been found by gender and ethnic group as well as social class. The NHS needs to do better on this equity of use criterion.

The third criterion is the most difficult to comment upon. Whilst 'the best' is still a matter for debate it is difficult to 'universalize' it. In some cases, however, it is at least feasible to make policy recommendations regarding 'the best'. There is evidence that cancer treatment outcomes are improved if treatment is given in highly specialized centres which have doctors and other staff familiar with the specific cancer type and site. These centres have a range of facilities for further investigations and treatment. However, even though a shift of treatment to such centres is an agreed policy aim of the NHS (the so-called 'Calman/Hine' policy) there is still an immense amount of work needed to achieve this.

These comments on equity, largely derived from Klein, require two further issues to be borne in mind. First, as Chapter 3 has shown, there remain large inequalities in health reflected by mortality and morbidity statistics. Second (as we will later argue), the NHS reforms have had a considerable adverse impact on the equity of access and use. The first of these issues illustrates the point that on its own an NHS equity strategy is ineffective, the second issue will require a further discussion later in this chapter. Anticipating, we might summarize that an equity strategy was not a political priority for the post-reform NHS in the period 1991–97.

Continuing the theme of rational planning versus 'muddling through' we can ask another deceptively simple question 'Is the NHS underfunded?' Answering this question, is said to be a 'metaphysical' endeavour (Klein). Others, however, take it to be at least partially open to a rational analysis and answer. In *The State of Welfare* (1989) the question is tackled by means of a statistical model. First, the actual expenditure on the NHS, measured in cash terms, is adjusted for inflation. The techniques for doing this vary. One method uses the 'GDP deflator', a measure of general inflation, this allows the calculation of 'real' expenditure in cash terms. However, price charges in the NHS may be very different relative to general inflation (the so-called relative price effect) so an 'NHS specific deflator' can be used to calculate the expenditure 'volume' – this index measures the amount of goods and services that can be bought at constant prices. Ageing of the population provides a crude measure of need, thus a demographic index of need can be calculated.

Table 6.1 is taken from *The State of Welfare* and shows expenditure (adjusted via the GDP deflator) and an expenditure volume index relative to a demographic need index for years 1973–87/8. This type of analysis has been updated in later work by Jennifer Dixon and colleagues.

The State of Welfare authors interpret these trends (to 1989) as follows. First, both Labour (1973/4 and 1978/9) and Conservative (1978/9–1987/8) administrations rapidly increased real expenditure shortly after they came to power. Labour increased real expenditure by over 20% in 1974/5, and Conservatives increased it by almost 10% in 1980/1. Generous pay awards seemed to explain both of these leaps in expenditure. In terms of the volume expenditure index, however, the trends show different patterns. The growth rate of resources going to the NHS under a Labour Government

Table 6.1: The National Health Service: growth in resources and needs

	Expenditures			
	£bn (real)	As % of GDP	Volume (1973/4 = 100)	Needs (1973/4 = 100)
1973/4	12.5	3.8	100	100
1974/5	15.1	4.6	113	100
1975/6	16.0	4.9	122	100
1976/7	16.1	4.8	123	100
1977/8	15.7	4.6	122	101
1978/9	16.1	4.5	124	101
1979/80	16.1	4.4	124	103
1980/1	17.7	5.0	130	104
1981/2	17.9	5.1	131	104
1982/3	18.1	5.1	133	105
1983/4	18.5	5.0	131	105
1984/5	18.7	4.9	133	106
1985/6	18.9	4.8	134	107
1986/7	19.7	4.8	133	108
1987/8	20.6[a]	4.9	n.a.	109

[a] Provisional.

Sources: Real expenditures: Table 4.A1; % of GDP: calculated from Table 4.A1 and CSO 1988b; volume: calculated from Table 4.A2; needs: *Official Report*, 26 March 1984, WA, col. 60, and *Official Report*, 23 June 1986, WA, col. 66–7.

was higher than under a Conservative Government. This prompts *The State of Welfare* authors to conclude

'Both governments can chalk up some policy successes over the period, particularly with respect to maintaining the overall level of resources .... There are differences between the governments, in particular, it is clear that the NHS was safer in the hands of Labour than it has been under Conservatives, at least so far as the volume of resources relative to need was concerned. However, the Conservative government has maintained the level of resources going to the NHS (and) has maintained a commitment to funding from general taxation ....'

Taking this analysis up to the year 1996/7 we can draw upon Jennifer Dixon and her colleagues' recent work. They show that both real expenditure and volume expenditure continued to increase faster than the need index based upon the ageing of the population. They further subdivide the expenditures into those going to Hospital and Community Services (HCS) and those going to the Family Health Services (FHS). In both of these sub-analyses the picture remained the same. With a few exceptions, funding increases remained faster than the index of need. One of the 'exceptions', however, occurs for the year 1996–97, the estimated real growth in spending on HCS for this year is 0.1%, but volume growth is estimated to be negative (–0.1%), this is a fall in the resources relative to needs. This explains the chorus of concern voiced by representatives of doctors (BMA) and managers of the service (National Association of Health Authorities and Trusts).

However, as all of those who have looked at the question of 'underfunding' know, the pressures on health services come from four principal sources: demographic change (principally ageing of the population), changes in the level of morbidity (e.g. a new disease like AIDS), technological innovations (e.g. 'keyhole' surgery) and, perhaps most important, changing expectations of both providers (doctors, nurses, etc.) and public. These 'cost drivers' have different levels of uncertainty and it is quite possible that technological progress and professional and public expectations regarding the application of technology could break the NHS 'bank'. Certainly, as Dixon and her colleagues argue, local management of hospital and community facilities can make a real difference in terms of the perception of 'underfunding'.

Considerations such as these draw one back to the absolute necessity of public involvement in priority setting within an informed and ethical framework (see Chapter 5). Technological 'fixes' in the future may deliver us from the burden of chronic diseases, but, as has been argued, we doubt it. Allowing technology changes to drive the NHS would be disastrous – there is always a slightly better machine or technique. Technologies must prove themselves through rigorous scientific evaluation (RCTs if feasible) and through marginal budgetary procedures (see Chapter 5). In the longer term, the reconfigured NHS (therapeutic outcome-led) will, we believe, have sufficient funds for effective therapies chosen through informed demands. As we suggested, the reconfiguration of the NHS depends primarily on an empowered public and a willingness by professionals to practise evidence-based medicine (or more widely evidence-based health care). These changes are quite feasible and the forces for change relatively strong.

The changes we desire in the social ideology of medicine are, however, more long term and will depend on the usefulness and truthfulness of our arguments about causation and the realist socio-political health policy it entails. How that story (biomedical vs socio-political models of health) will turn out is undecidable at this time. As we have said, our strong hunch is on a paradigm shift that will transform, among many other things, the teaching, learning and practice of clinical medicine. Just how such a transformation can be worked for within the current NHS will be outlined in Chapter 8, for now we must turn to the NHS as it has been and as it is, and develop a public health critique.

A public health NHS and a defence

The intellectual and conceptual resources for a public health critique of the current NHS have already been sketched out in this and previous chapters. Briefly, the NHS should reconfigure itself, separating, with some exceptions, 'cure' from 'care' services. Whilst a health professional leadership role is necessary in the cure service it is much less likely that this is so in the care service. Indeed, care services should be made much more open to other modes of service delivery, some involving and some not involving traditional health care practitioners. Care services standards should, however, be subject to licensing and accreditation by the state, both those with a reconfigured NHS and those in the private sector.

Private provision of care services, with consumers given adequate financial resources from the state, is both logical and ethically feasible, unlike the situation for cure services. No doubt opponents of this split will attempt to argue that 'cure' and 'care' are inseparable, or (amounting to the same thing) cannot be practically distinguished one from the other. This argument has force, but concerted attempts at drawing appropriate distinctions would, we believe, bear fruit. A conceptual and practical separation is possible.

Within the cure service the doctor–patient relationship should change to empower patients with relevant information so that both patient and doctor work as partners in a therapeutic alliance. Within the care service, consumers ('patient' is an inappropriate label here) are (very nearly) sovereign. The caveat is meant to serve as a reminder that in some cases this marketing imperative will be subject to ethical and, in some cases, health considerations.

But lest the critical tide we have summoned up in this and previous chapters threaten to engulf the NHS, it is, surely, time for a defence. The need for such a defence comes from a rational but naïve response to the criticisms made of the NHS. This attitude asks the question 'If the NHS fails in so many ways why bother with it?'

Images and historical understanding of pre-1948 (and especially pre-1939) life are one way to begin a defence. Medical care was available easily to those who could afford it, but others who were not covered by health insurance schemes worried about the cost. There was no pretence that health care was to be thought of as a right, which any and all people of the nation would have simply because they were citizens (or loyal subjects). The transformation of the relationship between people and the state forms the core of the work of TH Marshall. Marshall argued that the state first grants economic rights, then political rights and then, in a modern state, social rights. All of these are the outcomes of a struggle and are not to be discarded lightly.

Seen in this way the NHS, with its founding principles of equity and right, was a massive advance in the formation of a just and fair society. Richard Titmus, who was the first professor of social administration at the London School of Economics, has written movingly about the profound cultural importance of the NHS. Beyond its faults in making us all wait for treatment on waiting lists, losing our medical notes and exhorting us to do this or that, the NHS was 'our NHS'. In having such a national institution we rediscovered our social solidarity. Unlike the market, where we could get whatever we desired so long as we could pay the price, the NHS operated on what we needed, and we could expect our needs (or some of them) to be met whatever our poverty or wealth. The public's affection for the NHS is a constant finding in surveys of opinion. This affection reflects our continuing pride in an institution that strives to provide help and reassurance in times of adversity. Certainly, the NHS, from a cultural standpoint, is an achievement it is worth struggling to preserve.

But there are other arguments for the NHS. Though, as we have stated, the NHS has not been responsible for anything more than about 20% of the increase of life expectancy during the twentieth century this argument misses the point. As Rudolf Klein says, the argument is correct 'but vacuous'. Death rates (and life expectancy) though useful are blunt measures. What about the role of the NHS (and health care more generally) in restoring sight to those with cataracts, providing pain relief to those with arthritis, cancer and colic, mending broken bones, replacing worn out hips and so on and so on? The improvement in quality of life that accrues to such activities is unmeasured but is, without any doubt, substantial. Health services can contribute to care even if cure is not possible. The 'balance sheet' of the NHS (to use Klein's phrase) shows a profit.

Hardening the arguments still further there are sound reasons based on economic efficiency for the NHS and its founding principles. These principles, it will be recalled, are: services free at the point of use; comprehensive coverage of the population; funding, in the main, by means of general taxation. Nicholas Barr, in his book *The Economics of the Welfare State* (2nd edn, 1993), brings the economic arguments together. He discusses the NHS in comparison with three alternative systems that rely, respectively, on private provision and finance, public provision and insurance-based finance or private provision and public finance. He is able to conclude that the NHS fares better than alternative systems:

> The NHS thus has much to commend it; and many of its remaining problems could largely be resolved by giving it more resources and by gathering and using more and better information.

Moreover, though:

> No system of health care can be perfect – the real issue is to chose the best inefficient and inequitable form of organisation. Radical privatisation (private provision and private financing) is no way of doing so. This conclusion rests not on personal values but on the *technical* nature of health care, and particularly, though not exclusively, in information problems which are ignored in much of the pro-market literature.

The 'information problems' mentioned have been dealt with in previous chapters. Essentially, the mismatch in information between suppliers (health care professionals) and consumers (patients) means that the market assumptions that underpin private provision and private financing break down. In theory, privatization is not all-or-nothing. For instance, the NHS currently conforms to public provision (NHS facilities are publicly owned) with public financing (via general taxation), less than radical privatization would move one or other to the private sector. If, for example, private financing was to be pursued then a number of economic efficiency problems would arise. By describing these we can illustrate Barr's methods of argument.

If we each had to pay for our own health care we would, no doubt, seek to do so through some form of insurance. The real issue, then, is whether or not the private market can supply medical insurance efficiently. There are five technical conditions that must hold for any insurance scheme to be efficiently supplied by a market.

1 The probability of needing treatment must be independent across individuals.

2 This probability must be less than 1.

3 This probability must be known or be estimable.

4 There must be no substantial problem of *adverse selection*. This involves the supplier having as much information as the purchaser, so that the purchaser is unable to conceal facts about his or her health.

5 There must be no substantial problem of *moral hazard*. This occurs when the purchaser cannot (without incurring costs) manipulate the probability of the insured event (here the consumption of health care) without the supplier's knowledge.

Barr asks how far do these conditions hold for health care? The first condition breaks down because, as we have seen, certain characteristics of people do influence their probability (risk) of falling ill and hence of requiring treatment. These characteristics include age, occupational social class, economic activity, housing tenure and so on (see Chapter 3). The second condition holds for ill health following accidents and acute ill health, such as pneumonia or appendicitis, however, the risk of ill health associated with chronic conditions increases rapidly with increasing age, so much so that risk can approach 1. Thus the second condition breaks down. The third condition is possible because we can use epidemiological information to construct actuarial tables. Conditions 4 and 5 however are unrealistic for health care. Barr discusses adverse selection by quoting George Akerlof on the subject of why Americans aged over 65 cannot easily buy medical insurance. Akerlof concludes:

> ... that as the price of insurance rises the people who insure themselves will be those who are increasingly certain that they will need the insurance; for error in medical check-ups, doctors' sympathy with older patients, and so on make it much easier for the applicant to assess the risks involved than the insurance company.

On the final condition, absence of moral hazard, two general problems require attention: influence on consumption and cost of health care. First, patients who have full insurance cover may decide to take fewer preventive measures, thus altering upwards their disease risk. Also, all patients have the choice of consulting a doctor and have the choice over matters such as pregnancy – but these choices consume health care resources. Thus insured consumers can unilaterally influence the probability of consuming health care resources. Second, consumers of insurance can influence the cost of treatment. This is the so-called *third-party payment* problem. This problem arises because the patient and the health care provider can both act without regard to costs – they do not pay themselves, the insurance supplier picks up the bill. Typically then, this will lead to over consumption (and over treatment). Consequently insurance-based health care presents suppliers with insuperable technical difficulties.

Therefore, private insurance leads to gaps in coverage because suppliers will not take on certain risks (e.g. chronic illness, congenital illness, elderly) and inefficiency is likely due to the third-party payment problem. Though advocates of the market have devised schemes to lessen these problems, such as co-insurance, deductibles, compulsory participation via regulation, such solutions remain inadequate since they do not sufficiently repair the preconditions that should underpin private market provision. The NHS, it turns out, is supplied according to the theory of economic efficiency.

The reformed NHS (1991–97): better medicine?

The 1991 NHS reforms have already been described (Chapter 1) but we need to evaluate how successful or unsuccessful these organizational changes have been. The question of success, as we have seen, is not straightforward. In this area there are added difficulties because the NHS reform did not happen all at once, indeed changes were happening over an extended period of time. For example, general practice fundholding (GPFH) was originally allowed only for large practices (12 000 and over patients on the list) and GPFH status meant that budgets were given to the fundholder for a limited set of procedures. Originally, mental health services were excluded from the budget-holders remit as were a number of hospital procedures that were costly (over £6000). Later, however, list size to qualify for GPFH status was decreased (to 7000) and fundholders were allowed to hold budgets for more and more types of services. The pre-1997 General Election position was that fundholders were increasingly able to have 'total fundholding' status where they were allowed to hold a budget (including high-cost and emergency care). What, therefore, is the change that requires evaluation?

Further difficulties arise because in advocating reform the Department of Health came up with two rather vague policy objectives. These objectives were set out in the White Paper *Working for Patients*: first 'to give patients wherever they live in the UK, better health care and greater choice of services available', and second '[provide] greater satisfaction and reward for those working in the NHS who successfully respond to local needs and preferences'. Whilst it is possible to attempt to measure success or failure of the reforms in these terms there remain large problems of validity and reliability in the available data. How are we to operationalize the term 'better health care'? Certainly we can supply a public health answer to this – 'better' means effective and affordable health care that satisfies a health need, but measuring this achievement would require a major research study. In fact no research into the impact and outcomes of the NHS reforms was commissioned by the Department of Health (DoH) under the Conservative Government. It was left to independent charitable organizations to fund the meagre amount of research that was done. In the circumstances, one wonders if the DoH or anyone else in the former Government really wanted to know if the reforms had any effect, good or bad.

The research that does exist on the impact of the reforms routinely begins with a number of warnings and we have echoed these: the reforms were cumulative not one-off; attributing an outcome to the reforms themselves is very difficult (because trends were well in place prior to the reforms); and (even when we have clear-cut results) evaluation (specifying the change as 'good' or 'bad') is often impossible. As an example of the latter problem let's consider referrals from GPFH to hospital specialist (secondary) care. The existing research shows different things. Research on 'first wave' (i.e. early adopters) GPFHs in one English NHS Region showed no change in rates of referrals to hospital, however, research carried out in Scotland showed a significant decrease in referral rates. The point is how do we evaluate these findings: is 'no change' preferable to 'decrease' or vice versa?

If we attempt to eschew empirical evidence and go back to *a priori* theory we do no better. For example, GPFHs had economic incentives to 'make savings' in their spending because savings could be re-invested in developing their services or in upgrading the practice premises. However, the actual behaviour of GPs who were fundholders shows that in many cases no savings were made, in other cases savings were voluntarily paid back to the health authority and in other cases savings were re-used to upgrade premises – theory did not predict behaviour. This point is especially important because commentators on the NHS reforms have, in some cases, 'gone back to theory' to make evaluative points. One influential commentator, for instance, broadly welcomes the NHS internal market, even though it had very little similarity to a free market. It was claimed that the internal market remains theoretically attractive as health care is 'contestable'. By adjusting theory ever so slightly another influential commentator was able to make dire warnings about the impact of the reforms, again based on theory. These two commentaries appeared in the same book.

Certainly some things are clear. Transaction costs in the pre-1991 NHS were very low by international standards (perhaps around 4% of the NHS costs), after the reforms transaction costs were around three times as high. Competition in some areas was claimed to have improved operational efficiency. In direct pathology, for instance, some GPFH were successful in negotiating lower costs for tests. Their threat of going elsewhere paid off for them but it remains possible that it shifted the efficiency problem to other 'customers'. For example, if a local pathology service did not succeed in gaining contracts from the GPFH it might have had to increase costs for other users or go out of business. Surgery or intensive care without a local pathology service is not, however, a feasible option, so it would appear that efficiency gained in one part of the NHS (GPFH) would have been paid for by another part of the NHS (in-patient services).

It is also clear that the NHS reforms allowed a shift of power between consultants and GPs. This, again, requires evaluation. It is not obvious, for instance, whether quality of care was enhanced or diminished (or untouched) by this change. Certainly, from a long-cherished policy perspective this shift appears to be a 'good thing' since it (in theory) would allow GPs to intervene in more influential ways with specialists, safeguarding patients' interests. But, likewise, this power shift may have led to undertreatment or to over-treatment. The former would be predicted by economic theory (self-interest) and the latter by marketing theory (consultants making a pitch for customers). What did happen is an empirical question, which would have relied heavily on local circumstances.

Perhaps the most interesting finding regarding the post-reform NHS is the way that explicit regulation became a central part of the way services were provided. The political dilemma for all governments, it will be recalled, is that the state and performance of the NHS is seen as a responsibility of government, yet government is not in a position to control the NHS. The years 1991–97 saw an ever increasing regulation of the way the NHS internal market operated – quite against purist theory. Accountability reviews became a major feature of the hospital service and innovation in service delivery was remarkably slight. In respect of GPFH, the *Audit Commission* found that very little change had occurred or had been the result of fund-holding. Two forces appear to have been operating – bureaucratic regulation to stave off political gaffs (e.g. trust failures) and professional inertia.

Even with the vague objectives of increasing 'choice' and 'responsive-ness', the reforms are hard to evaluate. Choice was not increased for GPFH patients if patients did not make the relevant choices themselves. Given the nature of GPFH activities in the placing of 'cost–volume' contracts it was the GP, not the patient, who chose the hospital referral and chose the con-sultant. The responsiveness of the NHS is difficult to measure. If we try to use waiting times then we see that in some cases things improved and in others they did not. Responsiveness, measured in terms of patient satisfaction, also shows contradictory results. Turning to 'greater satisfaction' for pro-viders we also have mixed evidence. Some studies of GPFH showed that GPs did not regard fundholding as a positive voluntary choice, rather they felt they had been pushed into this choice in order to retain a degree of auto-nomy in the post-reform NHS. Consultants, too, voiced their dissatisfaction with their working conditions in trusts. On the other hand, many GPs working in fundholding practices felt they had more control over their work than in the pre-reform days.

From a public health medicine perspective one central feature of the NHS reforms requires further discussion – the purchaser–provider split. In theory, this should have allowed a more effective, efficient and equitable (the 3 Es) delivery of service. Public health doctors (with others) can ascertain the health care needs of their DHA population and advise on the most efficient mix of services, bearing in mind the need for equity. This appears to be a case where theory does have a useful role. Most public health doctors would, we suggest, retain the purchaser–provider split. However, it must be said that even if this division remains the problems of planning, let alone delivering a public health orientated mix of services, will remain daunting. The task of public health doctors in all of this remains the same: working with clinicians and managers to achieve the 3 Es.

Before leaving this discussion of the NHS reforms we need to recognize that these reforms contained within themselves certain contradictions. On the one hand, the policy objective was to improve choice and responsiveness yet it was the case that GPs, not patients, remained the choosers. Money did not 'follow patients', rather patients continued to follow the money. Moreover, there is evidence that trusts responded differently to GPFH-funded patients compared with patients referred from non-fundholding GPs. There is evidence that the former type of patients were given 'fast-track' service, with less waiting time for a specialist consultation. This practice made commercial sense (need to retain GPFH contracts) but is at odds with the NHS founding principle of equity. Though this practice received government disapproval the extent of its occurrence was unknown.

In the months before the 1997 General Election the future of the NHS was considered by both the Conservative Government and the opposition parties. There was a clear division between the Conservatives and Labour on a number of issues. Whereas Conservatives saw the reforms becoming consolidated and extended, especially in the area of primary care, Labour said it would undo key organizational relationships and 'end the internal market system'. Prior to the General Election no less than three White Papers were released in the space of six months. The purpose of these documents was to at once reaffirm that the NHS's founding principles would continue to underpin the service under a future Conservative Government and also to lay the foundations for a continuation of the shift in power, from hospital to primary care services.

The new slogan in these policy documents was the 'primary care-led NHS'. This vision sees GPs and other primary care staff taking on more and more roles, so that secondary care becomes less needed. Nurses, especially, were to be given an extended professional role that would include the ability to prescribe medicines from a limited list. GPs were to have their terms and conditions of service made more flexible and salaried GPs, de-livering services to the NHS, would be able to be employed by a number of employers. These employers might include hospitals or community trusts, or voluntary agencies or commercial enterprises. The purpose of these fur-ther reforms was couched in the now familiar formula of extending choice and the responsiveness of the NHS to patients. Whereas the first wave of reforms, as we have seen, did not in practice deliver these policy objectives the freeing up of the 'supply side' of medicine was seen as a potentially effective means to these ends.

What the likely outcome of this supply-side flexibility would have been is, as always, difficult to predict. In the sense that patient demands would have been more able to be effected (through greater choice of GP) there would have been an increase in choice and responsiveness. To this extent there would have been a real shift in power from supplier to consumer and this would have more closely mimicked a free-market system. However, as we have argued, health care has attributes that make it a non-tradable good. Foremost in this respect is the information gap. Freeing up supply, would, in itself, do nothing to remedy this. As demands are always likely to outstrip supply *given this information gap*, and because (in the absence of information regarding outcomes of therapies) demand is far greater than *need*, the NHS would have become a demand-led, rather than a need-led, organization. Waiting times would therefore have grown even if resource inputs matched historical levels. These levels of course, better reflected needs, not demands.

In such a situation it would have been likely that there would have been a continued exit from the NHS of those who could afford partic-ular types of private health care. Private health care insurance grew rap-idly in the 1980s and early 1990s. In 1997 around 12% of the population were privately insured. Consumption is mainly restricted to elective (non-emergency) surgery (such as hip replacements, hernia repair) and screening services (e.g. health checks, blood pressures, etc.). In some areas around one-third of elective hip replacements are paid for via private insurance.

The Labour Party, now the Government, came to power pledging the scrapping of hospital and community trusts and the ending of GPFH. Labour has also created the post of Minister for Public Health. Local health commissions will be formed, comprised of GPs and consultants, together with representatives from voluntary groups and members of the public.

Public health doctors will be included in these commissioning groups. The function of these groups will be to assess health care needs and commission services to meet the needs, where necessary prioritizing the needs and services commissioned.

Both Labour and Conservative Parties favour the retention of the purchaser–provider split, purchasing becoming 'commissioning' in the language of the Labour Party. Health authorities were to become, under both parties, more strategic. In the Conservative version of a primary care-led NHS, all GPs would have held budgets, so the health authority would not have money to spend, and (in the Labour version) local commissioning groups will be primarily responsible for spending. Thus, health authorities will be asked to become strategic authorities. How this will translate into organizational structures or function is, as yet, unclear.

What can we say about these developments? Public health medicine has a number of clear practical points that any reformer should attend to. These points arise out of both theory and the experience of planning, delivery and evaluation of health care services.

- The founding principles of the NHS are robust and should remain central in any further reforms.

- Health care systems must be designed to meet informed patient need *not* demands.

- Primary care should be resourced appropriately and the range and scope of services that are effectively, efficiently and acceptably provided at this level should be empirically determined.

- Primary care is not an appropriate setting for all types of service.

- Empowerment of patients should become a basic objective of all health care.

- Research must continue and be expanded so that the scientific status and costs of therapies is known and better means of providing professional and patient education on effectiveness issues should be found.

- Cure services might be usefully separated from care services, with the latter allowed an expanded range of provision and organizational form, subject to quality standards.

- Research into the social, economic and political causes of disease and health (public health research) should be supported and the scope of interdisciplinary funding expanded.

These recommendations add up to our version of a reconfigured NHS. Whether the current vision for the NHS on offer from politicians will forward this agenda remains, as ever, speculative. The founding principles of the NHS are robust and further reform should enable their achievement. We emphasize that any reform must be part of a much greater effort to bring about a realist health policy and it is this issue which we take up in the next chapter.

Case study

Maintaining equity in the NHS

Earlier in the chapter, we briefly reviewed the equity considerations described by Aneurin Bevan – the equity of economic access, of geography and thirdly of use. Let us consider each of these in a little more detail, particularly in the context of attempting to maintain the different types of equity in the NHS of today and the future.

We suggested that the equity of economic access had, overall, been achieved. We need to remember, however, that increasingly over the last two decades health authorities were (with some difficulty, it must be said) creating policies whereby some treatments were of lower priority than others (Chapter 5). Frequently, this resulted in patients being required to pay for these procedures, e.g. treatments for infertility and cosmetic surgery being sought in the private sector and, often perversely, being provided by the same doctor who might have treated them without charge in the NHS. Moreover, whilst it is undoubtedly true that charges for prescriptions and some services are not levied on vulnerable groups, it is increasingly found that the prescription charge is at such a level to actually deter some patients from proceeding with their treatment. We should add that in a further group of treatments, comprising complementary therapies, some can be accessed and are available (on a highly selected and seemingly arbitrary basis) within the NHS, whilst the same therapies in other areas may not be available, with patients being required to obtain them privately.

We also considered geographical inequities and suggested that the NHS had performed less well, quoting Julian Tudor-Hart's 'inverse care law'. In the King's Fund publication *Tackling Inequalities in Health* (1996), the authors note that evidence about equitable access to care in Britain is patchy. They comment that on the one hand there is some evidence that implies that the NHS does surprisingly well in ensuring that resources are distributed between social groups in proportion to their relative needs. On the other hand, the authors note that a number of small scale studies suggest that among a range of specific services and at local levels, more disadvantaged social groups appear to be under-served. Consequently, in these instances geographical inequity is produced through a social class inequity in access.

As we have previously said, universalizing the best services (the third type of equity) will require a substantial amount of work. Attempts to define the best services are now well under way through international, national, and regional R&D programmes, clinical effectiveness initiatives and the comparison of 'best practice' with local services (clinical audit). Although concerted attempts are now underway to ensure that the best care is delivered to specific patient groups, e.g. referral of cancer patients to accredited cancer units and/or cancer centres, this has involved an enormous amount of effort from a very wide range of health professionals and users. Is a similar effort warranted for other prioritized services in, for example, *The Health of the Nation* national strategy? We think this issue requires a wide-ranging debate to agree an appropriate programme of service development, which includes the whole spectrum of health care, i.e. prevention, diagnosis and rehabilitation.

Issues surrounding equity of use can only, we feel, be dealt with in the short term by appropriate financial resourcing of the NHS, but as we have already discussed, this is a debate which must not only involve the health professionals but a public which is, at best, informed and, at least, involved. Tackling and maintaining equity of geographical use is, we feel, best undertaken by local commissioning, which will involve health needs analysis at a localized level followed, hopefully, by appropriate commissioning of health care to meet those needs. Increasingly, the drive towards a more primary care-based NHS will allow a better and, hopefully, effective delivery of appropriate care locally.

Notes

The NHS is fertile ground for policy analysis. See, for example, Chris Ham's book *Management and Competition in the New NHS* (Oxford: Radcliffe Medical Press, 1994) and Ray Robinson and Julian Le Grand (eds) *Evaluating the NHS Reforms* (London: King's Fund Institute, 1994), A Culyer *et al.* (eds) *Competition in Health Care: Reforming the NHS* (London: Macmillan, 1990), Steven Harrison, David Hunter and Chris Pollitt's *The Dynamics of British Health Policy* (London: Unwin Hyman, 1900), and Rudolf Klein's

The Politics of the NHS (London: Longman, 1989), for a variety of views. The book *The State of Welfare: The Welfare State in Britain since 1974* is edited by John Hills (Oxford: Clarendon Press, 1990). For an updating of their analysis of 'underfunding' see, Jennifer Dixon and Anthony Harrison's article 'Funding in the NHS – A little local difficulty?' (*BMJ*. 1997; **314**: 216–19). For Richard Titmuss' views of the NHS see, *The Problems of Social Policy* (London: HMSO, 1950), *Essays on 'The Welfare State'* (London: Allen and Unwin, 1958) and especially, *Commitment to Welfare* (London: Allen and Unwin, 1968). The economic argument for the NHS is found in Nicholas Barr's book *The Economics of the Welfare State* (Oxford: Oxford University Press, 2nd edn, 1993). George Akerlof's article is 'The Market for "Lemons": Qualitative Uncertainty and Market Mechanism' (*Quarterly Journal of Economics*. 1970; **84**: 488–500).

7

A policy for health?

The annual *State of the Public Health in England* report is the place where the Chief Medical Officer (CMO) provides a summary of the public health issues that are deemed important enough for official comment. In this report for 1995 there is this valedictory passage:

> The Government's strategy for health in England was launched in July 1992 in the *Health of the Nation* White Paper. This innovative initiative to improve the health of the entire population focused on five key areas responsible for much of the avoidable ill-health and premature death in England, and set out to redress the balance between health care (the treatment of ill-health) and health promotion – the preservation of good health and the development of better health.

The *Health of the Nation* is the name given to a policy launched by the former Conservative Government which aimed to improve the health of the people in England. Other countries (Wales, Scotland, Northern Ireland) also had their own policies which, though differing in detail, shared a basic underpinning philosophy with the English policy. Two central features of these policies are:

1 They all identify key areas for health improvement, set target objectives and aim to monitor their achievement.

2 They all rely on a behaviour modification strategy as the central means of achieving disease prevention and health promotion.

These features are placed within a policy that announces that health and disease are the outcome of a complex interplay of influences. The Green Paper (1991), for example, clearly recognized this reality in affirming

> ... that as health is determined by a whole range of influences – from genetic inheritance, through personal behaviour, family and social environment – so opportunity and responsibilities for action to improve health are widely spread from individuals to Government as a whole.

This chapter will examine the *Health of the Nation (HoN)* policy in the light of the realist health policy framework sketched out in previous chapters. It should be said immediately that the intention of this analysis is not to score ideological points or judge this health policy useless. We will claim that the *Health of the Nation* was a pragmatic compromise constructed within a social and political environment which would not have been receptive to a radical health policy. We will also claim, however, that this conservatism will now require a radical transformation if the aim of a national policy for health – maintaining and improving health for all – is to be realized. We begin by describing the policy, we then critically examine it against a realist policy and conclude by sketching out problems that a realist (socio-political) health policy must resolve.

The Health of the Nation

Announcing the key areas of the health policy for England the White Paper (1992) explains that they were chosen because they were areas where 'there is both the greatest need and greatest scope for making cost-effective improvements in the overall health of the country'. The five key areas are:

1 Coronary heart disease and stroke

2 Cancers (breast, cervical, lung)

3 Mental illness

4 HIV/AIDS and sexual health

5 Accidents

This initial selection was chosen from 16 possible areas that were discussed in the consultation Green Paper (1991), these areas included: health of pregnant women, infants and children; diabetes; food safety; rehabilitation services for people with a physical disability; asthma; environment and health. The White Paper mentions in passing why such areas were left out of the announced policy. For instance, maternal and child health, food safety and oral health were left out because these were areas 'with existing initiatives which are sufficiently well developed not to require the status of a Key Area …' In passing, we can say that the bovine spongiform encephalopathy (BSE)/food hygiene problems since 1992 make this official sentiment at the very least complacent. Environment and health as a key area has been the subject of a consultation exercise prior to its introduction. This consultation has generally been favourable but the intended targets show two glaring omissions – missing are targets for PM_{10} (particulate air pollution) and improved housing conditions (particularly regarding space and avoidance of indoor damp). It is to be hoped that these targets will be included in a future specification.

Within each key area adopted objectives were identified and targets were set. It was considered necessary to set targets because they would 'give a clarity to the objectives, allow different groups to focus on the common objective and provide a *yardstick for measuring achievement*'. Box 7.1 summarizes the objectives and targets of the health policy.

The way to achieve these objectives was given only a brief treatment in the White Paper. In essence, it was emphasized that responsibilities for achievement were diffuse; individuals, professional health workers, voluntary agencies, government agencies (especially the NHS and Department of Health) all had roles to play. Strategic direction would be given from the centre (DoH, NHS Executive) but implementation was to be a local task. The idea of bringing agencies together to form voluntary *Health Alliances* was given pride of place in the White Paper. Moreover certain settings such as cities, schools, hospitals and prisons were exhorted to involve themselves in health promotion activities and become *Healthy Cities, Healthy Schools* and so on. Many of these settings were already sites for health promotion activities. The WHO, for example, had set up a Healthy City Network during the 1980s and the intention of the government was to build on these initiatives not replace them.

The role of the government was seen as: 'a facilitator of change, a source of legislation and regulation, information and monitoring and an allocator of resources'. An important point was the role of government in co-ordinating policy from different departments. The White Paper stated:

> Many policies have, to a greater or lesser degree, an impact on health. It is important, therefore, that as policy is developed the consequences for health are assessed and, where appropriate, taken into account. **The government will produce guidance on 'policy appraisal and health'** – a similar approach to guidance on 'policy appraisal and the environment' which was produced following publication of the Environment White Paper 'This Common Inheritance'. (emphasis in the original)

The monitoring of target achievement would be at national level. For many targets the data would be available from existing surveys but for some, notably for coronary heart disease and mental illness, new surveys were planned.

Box 7.1: Health of the Nation main targets

Coronary heart disease and stroke:

- To reduce the death rate for both CHD and stroke in people under 65 by at least 40% by the year 2000 (*Baseline 1990*)

- To reduce the death rate for CHD in people aged 65–74 by at least 30% by the year 2000 (*Baseline 1990*)

- To reduce the death rate for stroke in people aged 65–74 by at least 40% by the year 2000 (*Baseline 1990*)

Cancers:

- To reduce the death rate for breast cancer in the population invited for screening by at least 25% by the year 2000 (*Baseline 1990*)

- To reduce the incidence of invasive cervical cancer by at least 20% by the year 2000 (*Baseline 1986*)

- To reduce the death rate for lung cancer under the age of 75 by at least 30% in men and by at least 15% in women by 2010 (*Baseline 1990*)

- To halt the year-on-year increase in the incidence of skin cancer by 2005

Mental illness:

- To improve significantly the health and social functioning of mentally ill people

- To reduce the overall suicide rate by at least 15% by the year 2000 (*Baseline 1990*)

- To reduce the suicide rate of severely mentally ill people by at least 33% by the year 2000 (*Baseline 1990*)

HIV/AIDS and sexual health:

- To reduce the incidence of gonorrhoea by at least 20% by 1995 (*Baseline 1990*), as an indicator of HIV/AIDS trends

- To reduce by at least 50% the rate of conceptions amongst the under 16s by the year 2000 (*Baseline 1989*)

Accidents:

- To reduce the death rate for accidents among children aged under 15 by at least 33% by 2005 (*Baseline 1990*)

- To reduce the death rate for accidents among children aged 15–24 by at least 25% by 2005 (*Baseline 1990*)

- To reduce the death rate for accidents among people aged 65 and over by at least 33% by 2005 (*Baseline 1990*)

Before we assess *The Health of the Nation* policy we need first to note some issues concerning behaviour modification and inequalities in health. Behaviour modification approaches to preventive medicine and health promotion were outlined in Chapter 3. The patient is seen as either those with high risk of disease or as everyone in a population. The technologies available for behaviour modification are based on one or other model of *health education*, where individuals (either alone or with their family or others) decide to modify their behaviour by eliminating unhealthy activities and replacing them with healthy behaviours. The *HoN* main targets in the key areas are written as *outcome* targets, i.e. 'To reduce death rates by … ', and outcome targets are to be achieved, in large part, through *behaviour modification* targets (called risk factor targets in *HoN* documents), see Box 7.2.

Inequalities in health are not mentioned in the Green or White Paper, the term used is *variations in health*. These variations are briefly described within each key area and general statements are occasionally made. For example, in an appendix which discusses particular groups (elderly people, women, people from black and ethnic minority groups) there is a sub-heading *socio-economic group*. This brief note begins 'In England, as in all other westernised countries, there are variations in health status between different socio-economic groups within the population'. This variation is probably due to '… a complex interplay of genetic, biological, social, environmental, cultural and behavioural factors'. Targets for reducing health inequalities are not set.

Assessing the *Health of the Nation*

On its publication the *HoN* received a mixed press. On the whole, professionals within public health welcomed the strategy because it represented the first national strategic statement concerning health rather than health care in the history of the NHS. The missing issues of health inequalities, intersectoral policy development and resources for the strategy were sometimes noted by reviewers but a conscious effort seems to have been made to accentuate the positive. From a tactical view point criticism of the *HoN* and related policies in Wales, Scotland and Northern Ireland was deemed to be counterproductive.

There appeared at first to be scope within the policy for radical reforms, e.g. targeting inequalities in health. However, the history of *HoN* shows that these types of change did not occur. The reasons for this reflect the familiar catalogue displayed in Chapter 6. Specifically, there was a national 'enterprise

Box 7.2: Health of the Nation risk factor targets

Smoking:

- To reduce the prevalence of cigarette smoking to no more than 20% by the year 2000 in both men and women (a reduction of a third) (*Baseline 1990*)

- To reduce consumption of cigarettes by at least 40% by the year 2000 (*Baseline 1990*)

- In addition to the overall reduction in prevalence, at least 33% of women smokers to stop smoking at the start of their pregnancy by the year 2000

- To reduce smoking prevalence of 11–15 year olds by at least 33% by 1994 (to less than 6% (*Baseline 1988*)

Diet and nutrition:

- To reduce the average percentage of food energy derived by the population from saturated fatty acids by at least 35% by 2005 (to no more than 11% of food energy) (*Baseline 1990*)

- To reduce the average percentage of food energy derived from total fat by the population by at least 12% by 2005 (to no more than about 35% of total food energy) (*Baseline 1990*)

- To reduce the proportion of men drinking more than 21 units of alcohol per week and women drinking more than 14 units per week by 30% by 2005 (to 18% of men and 7% of women) (*Baseline 1990*)

Blood pressure:

- To reduce mean systolic blood pressure in the adult population by at least 5 mmHg by 2005 (*Baseline to be derived from new national health survey*)

HIV/AIDS:

- To reduce the percentage of injecting drug misusers who report sharing injecting equipment in the previous 4 weeks from 20% in 1990 to no more than 10% by 1997 and no more than 5% by the year 2000 culture' in the wake of the Thatcher years and though the times were thought to have become less 'Me' oriented and more 'caring', clearly local health policy-makers did not see this as opening an opportunity for a fundamental shift in health policy. Moreover, too many organizational changes had been set in motion by the NHS reforms. This made the centre (DoH) anxious to manage change and, as we have discussed, paradoxically given the rhetoric of responsiveness to local needs, the new health authorities were given strong directives about how to deal with a large list of topics. In this culture and organizational environment basic reorientation of health policy came very low on anyone's agenda.

The targets formed the backbone of a *management by objectives* framework, though how to attain these targets was, and remains, rather mysterious. The behaviour modification targets, for instance, were not always calculated to deliver the required decrease in death rates. In coronary heart disease for instance, decreases in the saturated fat content of diets, decreased obesity, decreased smoking and decreased systolic blood pressure would not together yield the 40% reduction in death rates required for men aged less than 65. However, it appears that what would yield this decrease is the continuation of a trend that had become established in England since 1979. The reasons for this trend are still a matter for speculation. Certainly reduced smoking prevalence will have contributed but this has accompanied increased prevalence of obesity and no discernible decrease in mean blood cholesterol levels (since 1991).

The target of a 40% reduction in stroke rate for those aged 65–74 (from baseline 1990) by the year 2000 is more firmly grounded in the relationship between blood pressure levels and risk of stroke. A 5 mmHg reduction in systolic blood pressure would yield a 40% reduction in stroke death rates. However, the former target is timed for 2005 whereas the latter is to be achieved by the year 2000. Since 1990 there has been a fall in stroke mortality rate of 14.3% (to 1995), a rate of decrease of 2.8% per year. On this rate of fall the target will not be hit (28.3 vs 40%). Once again, however, this analysis gives way to that based on extrapolation of time trends established in England since at least 1970. On these trends a 40% reduction appears to be comfortably achievable. Certainly we cannot tie this favourable trend in stroke mortality to a trend in decreased mean systolic blood pressure. The little evidence of the latter shows it is far too small to account for the former.

In making these observations regarding the processes probably involved in target setting we need to reiterate that they are not primarily meant as criticisms. Setting out predictions for the future based on what has occurred in the past is nothing new. Financial analysts ('chartists') use this method – called 'chartism' – to predict fluctuations in the stock market. Looking at the trends in disease mortality rates and setting targets on the basis of these trends is a reasonable thing to do given the need to show success in achieving targets. This need for success is only partly self-serving for the civil servants, policy-makers and politicians who constructed *HoN*. Whilst achievement of targets is seen, and is used, as an unquestionable justification of the policy, another use is to raise morale among NHS workers and this is no bad thing.

Within the achievable national targets, however, lies another, and more important story, the continuing tale of inequalities in health. The *HoN*, as we have seen, acknowledged variations in health as a fact but declined to make them a central objective for policy action. There was no target for reduction in inequalities and it is this fact that distinguishes *HoN* from its intellectual and institutionalized forerunner, the *Health for All By The Year 2000 (HFA)* policy of the World Health Organization (WHO).

The *HFA 2000* policy was developed in response to a ground-breaking resolution passed at the 30th World Health Assembly meeting (the governing body of the WHO) in 1977. This resolution stated:

> ...the main social target of Governments and WHO in the coming decades should be the attainment by all citizens of the world by the year 2000 of a level of health that will permit them to lead a socially and economically productive life.

The European Region of the WHO pursued this common goal by officially adopting 38 targets for health that were published in 1985 as a Health Policy for Europe. The first of these 38 targets is as follows:

> By the year 2000, the actual differences in health status between countries and between groups within countries should be reduced by at least 25 percent, by improving the level of health of disadvantaged nations and groups.

Six themes are used to ground and organize the health targets and it is useful to set these out in full.

Equity

Everyone should have an equal opportunity of obtaining and maintaining good health such that inequalities in health either between or within nations is abolished.

Health promotion

This recognizes the importance of preventing disease and promoting a healthy lifestyle; moreover a positive sense of health is seen as a necessary goal for health policy.

Community participation
Each person has responsibility for his or her health and should share this responsibility with health care workers and others. Crucially, people need to have sufficient information to take an active role in shaping their health.

Multi-sectorial co-operation
The health sector is only one of many sectors that must collaborate in promoting and maintaining health and preventing disease. Healthy public policy is a vital part of ensuring health promotion.

Primary health care
The basic health needs of people should be met by providing care as close as possible to where people live and work, such care must be readily accessible and acceptable to each local community.

International co-operation
Because health problems are international there must be a sharing of knowledge, experience and expertise with others in the fight against disease, illness and disability.

These themes form the backbone of a wide-ranging approach to health policy development and would facilitate what we have referred to as a socio-political or realist health policy. The importance of making equity a central theme of health policy emphasizes the epidemiological lessons which show inequalities to be causal mechanisms for ill-health. The role of public policy is explicitly acknowledged in target 13:

> By 1990, national policies of all Member States should ensure that legislature, administrative and economic mechanisms provide broad intersectoral support and resources for the promotion of healthy life-styles and ensure effective participation of the people at all levels of such policy-making.

Lifestyle is here seen as one part of the picture and the social, political and economic context of lifestyles is the other part. Consequently, in *HFA 2000* changing lifestyles is not seen as an individualized problem of choice, it is seen as being obstructed or facilitated by its inseparable environmental context. Choosing to eat more healthily, for example, is not unreasonably seen as dependent on the availability of economic resources to pay the higher prices required to purchase the healthy foods.

Another policy forerunner of *HoN* is the series of health policy statements made by the United States Surgeon General (roughly equivalent to the Chief Medical officers in the UK Government). Starting in 1979 with *Healthy People* the US health policy for the 1980s was set in train. National health promotion and disease prevention objectives were set and have since been updated for the 1990s in the current health policy *Healthy People 2000*. This policy was started in 1990 and is organized around three *Goals for the Nation*. These goals are said to '...permeate the structure and content of this report'.

They further define the challenge, especially for health planners, policy-makers and providers:

'Increase the span of healthy life for Americans
Reduce health disparities among Americans
Achieve access to preventative services for all Americans'.

Like *HFA 2000* the US health policy sets quantified targets for disease prevention. In contrast to *HoN*, the US policy also sets targets for reducing health inequalities (disparities) in the major disease categories.

Taking all of this into account the *HoN* policy can be seen, and we believe it was seen, as a pragmatic solution to the need for a national policy of health promotion in the context of *HFA 2000*. Times, as we have noted, were not conducive to an emphasis on health inequalities and, in any case, it might be argued that decreased disease rates were a good thing however they were achieved. A decrease is, after all, a decrease. We should not, how-ever, accept this latter argument from a public health perspective. A de-crease in the overall rate may be achieved in the face of either no change or an adverse change in a subgroup. Certainly our earlier discussion of Rawlsian justice ought to make us sensitive to this possibility and, if it were found to be the case, spur action to redress the injustice.

Such a situation of overall improvement masking a worsening of a subgroup is in fact found in male mortality rate in England and Wales.* For men as a whole, all-cause mortality rate improved over the 20-year period 1970–72 to 1991–93, from 573 to 424 deaths for every 100 000 men (a 26% decrease). This period saw mortality rates for social class I men decrease by 36%, but for men in social class V the same period saw an increase of 2% in mortality rate. Though overall male life expectancy has continued to im-prove (from 71.03 years in 1982 to 73.58 years in 1992), for men aged 25–39 life expectancy actually fell – this is the first time this has happened during the twentieth century.

---

* At the time of writing comparable data for Scotland and Northern Ireland were not available.

Death rates for suicide and lung cancer show a four-fold and five-fold difference, respectively, for social class V compared with social class I and social class gradients remain a major feature for the majority of diseases. If we turn to behaviour modification we can see similar differences between overall trends and subgroup trends. The decrease in cigarette smoking in England and Wales between 1975 and 1990 saw smoking rates halve (from 40% to 20%) among households in the upper quarter of income distribution.

However, among households in the lowest quarter of income, smoking rate remained at 51%. Among lone-parent households the smoking rate remained at 60% during this period. The explanation for these findings given by the study authors is deliberately understated; it appears that 'smoking is used as an anodyne against living on benefits'. We should remember that the current (1995) level of smoking among women in social class I is 22% and among women in social class V it is 36% (see Table 3.1). Moreover, there is evidence that this difference is due to more social class V women starting smoking rather than more social class I women quitting. Given this, it is worrying that there is evidence that over the last few years more teenage girls have taken up smoking. This makes the original *HoN* target on smoking practically unattainable (see Box 7.2). The Labour Government's commitment to banning all tobacco advertising and sponsorship is likely to help get this target back on track but it remains unlikely that the original target date will be met.

Summing up our criticisms of the *HoN* we will reiterate two points. First, there is an overemphasis on a behaviour modification approach. This sees health behaviour as individually chosen and individually modifiable by personal choice. Our previous discussion (Chapter 3) challenges these assumptions, and a recent study of childhood accidents adds to this criticism. Between 1985 and 1992 child deaths from injury (ages 0–14) declined by 35% in England and Wales. However, this decrease was accompanied by substantial decreases in average distances walked or cycled by children. The authors conclude that: 'A substantial proportion of the decline in pedestrian traffic and pedal cycling deaths … seems to have been achieved at the expense of children's walking and cycling activities. Changes in travel patterns may exact a considerable price in terms of future health problems'. Inactivity may well add to the burden of coronary heart disease and osteoporosis in future years, and will immediately add to the growing problem of childhood obesity and have an impact on psycho-social development. Consequently, one target (child accidents) is bought for the price of another health goal (though not a current *HoN* target), reducing childhood obesity. However, the strong relationship between child and adult obesity makes attainment of the target on the latter remote. Indeed, adult obesity prevalence is currently increasing. The message for health planners can be spelled out as follows: individual level behaviour must be seen in a wider social and environmental context. Failure to see this wider picture makes it likely that behaviour modification alone is unlikely to deliver sustainable improvements in health.

The second criticism is that by not making inequalities in health a theme that gives structure to the policy (as in *HFA 2000* and *Healthy People 2000*) the attainment of overall targets is likely to mask growing inequalities in health, a situation that defies social justice and the espoused goal of the NHS.

On the positive side, the *HoN* has put health promotion and disease prevention on the NHS and Whitehall's agenda. It is achieving many of its targets (whatever one's view of their origin) and it is still possible that the *HoN* key areas and targets can be modified to encompass a realist health policy. If this were done, the prime health goal would be restated: To reduce inequalities in health by improving the health of the worst off and effecting the promotion of health for all.

Unequal Britain

The realization that inequalities in health not only mirror social and economic inequalities, but that improving health for all can be achieved by reducing these inequalities marks a paradigm shift for public health and politics. The discourse of politics has been, until now, concerned with matters of social justice, seen primarily as the answers given to the questions 'who gets what?' and 'who decides and how do they decide?' Arguments for equality have always been based on ethical and economic arguments. This traditional discourse must now make room for the causal role that these inequalities have on health. Discussions about poverty have been derailed by the seemingly insoluble problems of definition (what is the 'poverty line'?) but the evidence shows that within countries it is *relative* rather than *absolute* poverty that explains health inequalities (see Chapter 3). It is this fact that can, and should, transform the terms of the traditional debate on poverty and health.

In what follows we briefly discuss the fault lines of contemporary inequality in England and Wales. The health policy response is to tackle inequalities head on and to see inequalities as connected with each other through the life-chances available to individuals and families. These problems form an interconnected web and should be understood in this way rather than as isolated social problems. Inevitably, we cannot include all the areas of inequality here, but those we have chosen illustrate the scale of the problem.

Poverty

Peter Townsend's book *A Poor Future* (1996) presents officially collected statistics that show poverty in Britain to have increased over the last two decades. In 1979 there were 860 000 children living in households with incomes below the middle of the income range for the poorest 10% of the population; in 1992–93 (latest available) this figure had risen to 1 180 000. These figures are for households after they have paid housing costs and are not due to increases in the child population. Over this period the child population actually declined. For adults too, there has been an increase of those living at this level of poverty: 2 000 000 in 1979 and 2 970 000 in 1992–93. If one draws the poverty line at 50% of the 1979 average income, then in 1979 there were 3 850 000 adults and 1 430 000 children and in 1992–93 there were 4 100 000 adults and 1 940 000 children living in poverty. That is one in every four people was living in poverty according to the 'official' measure used to characterize 'low income' (official statistics do not refer to 'poverty').

During this period the poorest section of the population did worse in absolute terms. In 1979, a married couple with two children aged three and eight would have had a disposable income (after housing costs) of £106 per week (at 1995 prices). This family (living in the poorest 10% of the income distribution) saw their disposable income reduced by £18 per week by 1992–93.

These statistics are borne out by qualitative research published by the Joseph Rowntree Foundation as *Life on a Low Income* (1996). This covered 31 studies and showed that an extra £15 per week income would make a great deal of difference for these households. This is the amount that benefits would have been uprated by if the link with average earnings had not been stopped in 1980. In a 'minimal essential budget' (which included items generally considered as essential and chosen at their cheapest prices) constructed for a child aged two to five years it was found that Income Support plus family premium (1994 rates) supplied only £20.68 per week of the £30.73 needed for a girl or the £32.25 needed for a boy.

Income inequality

The extent of income inequality is, like poverty, causally related to the distribution of disease and ill health. Inequality in income has increased since

1979 and, according to A.B. Atkinson: 'This widening of income differences is a departure from the pattern of previous decades in the UK which saw a modest reduction in income inequality over the post-war period'. The extent and trend of income inequality can be measured by means of the Gini coefficient. This is an index which would take the value of zero if all incomes were identical and would approach 100% if all income was received by one person.

Up to 1977 income inequality in the UK fell, and the Gini coefficient decreased from 26 in 1970 to 16 in 1977. From 1978–79, however, there has been a steady rise in this coefficient, rising by nearly nine points until 1991. This rise is more than double the decline in the UK that occurred between 1949 and 1976. Indeed, the rise in UK income inequality during the 1980s far outpaces the pattern seen in other countries: Australia, Japan and the US showed a 2–3 percentage point increase, whilst Canada and Ireland showed no upward trend during this period and Sweden showed a 4 percentage point rise in income inequality. In the UK, the rise in income inequality was especially striking during the second half of the 1980s: the Gini coefficient rising from 24.8 in 1979 to 27.9 in 1985, and rising to 33.7 in 1991.

For the poorest tenth of the population real average income after housing costs decreased by 17% between 1979 and 1992/93 whilst for the whole population the average income increased by 38%. These trends meant that a single adult, in the poorest tenth, had lost £364 per year by 1992/93, whilst a single adult in the richest tenth had gained £5,824 (April 1995 prices).

Employment

There are two issues regarding employment: level and security of employment. Both unemployment and insecure employment have an effect on health status and risk of disease. Moreover, the conditions under which people work, including psychological and social conditions, influence disease risk. Whilst claimant unemployment levels are declining in the UK there appears to be changes in the structure of the labour market that have increased insecurity of employment. Commentators cite three components of job insecurity: the level of protection enjoyed; the likelihood of losing one's job; and the degree of hurt and loss that results from being made redundant.

A measure of the first component is those in full-time employment with sufficient tenure to be covered by basic employment rights legislation. In 1975, this stood at 56% of the working age population, in June 1996 it was

36%. On the second component we can look at two measures: median job tenure and likelihood of losing a job measured by the probable number of jobs held over a lifetime. In 1975, the median job tenure for men was 99 months, in 1994 it was 73 months. However, for women these figures were 46 and 54 months respectively, indicating that women were, on average, becoming more secure in jobs while men were becoming less secure. The probable number of jobs over a lifetime for men and women was 6.75 in 1975 but rose to 8.5 in 1993.

The third component (hurt and loss due to redundancy) can be approached by considering the likely fate of anyone made redundant. Benefits whilst out of work have fallen relative to wages and are time limited. It is also known that the average wage earned by those who re-enter employment after a spell of unemployment is around £110 per week (1996 prices), which is less than half the average weekly wage for all jobs. Moreover, re-entry jobs are more likely to be part-time or temporary (60%) compared with all jobs (25%). There is another aspect to the question of employment concerning the workforce available for work. In the first quarter of 1996 the number of people with jobs fell by 74 000, but the unemployment rate also declined because the workforce (defined as those in employment plus those who want to work and qualify for benefit) fell even more. People leaving the workforce may do so in a variety of ways: early retirement, becoming incapacitated and disabled or simply discontinuing to claim Job Seeker's Allowance and living off savings or entering the unofficial ('black') economy. All these categories, plus those who want to work but believe there is no chance of finding a job (so-called 'discouraged workers'), make up those who are officially classified as 'economically inactive'. Certainly there has been a massive increase in those disabled and claiming Invalidity Benefit (IVB). This jumped from 400 000 in 1970 to 1.4 million in 1992 and the rise prompted the replacement of IVB by Incapacity Benefit in 1996. This new benefit comes with a much tightened 'all-work test' which now acts as a gatekeeper to this benefit.

For those remaining in the workforce the 1980s and 1990s has seen a huge rise in poorly paid jobs, the so-called atypical types of work: part-time, temporary and contract work, and a large rise in self-employment. Part-time work rose from 3.3% of all male employment in 1982 to 6.7% in 1993; for women these figures were 42.4 and 45.5%, respectively. Evidence from a survey conducted in 1995 shows that 'involuntary' part-time work (done because full-time work was unavailable) accounts for 27% of male part-time work and around one-tenth of the female part-time work. This type of work has a high turnover in males and in older females. As stated, currently 60% of all new jobs are part-time. Temporary work includes seasonal, casual or intermittent work and interim contracts through a temporary employment agency. This type of work accounted for 4.3% of male and 6.4% of female employment in 1986 and 6.2% and 7.8%, respectively, in 1995. Involuntary temporary work was reported by 52% of males and 38% of females in 1995. Self-employment grew from 6.6% in 1982 to 13% (18% in males, 7% in females) in the UK in 1990. The growth of these types of employment have major implications for current poverty, the viability of the welfare state in future years and for the level of low-incomes and poverty among future pensioners.

Housing

Perhaps the most visible symbol of the state of society during the 1980s and 1990s is the person sleeping on the street. An official census of rough sleepers in 1991 estimated that there were 2650 in England, 32 in Wales and 145 in Scotland. These figures, however, are considered a major underestimate by most experts. More reliably, the characteristics of rough sleepers (who may also at times use direct access hostels, night shelters and B&B hotels) were reported in 1993. Of those attending soup runs (and therefore more likely to be sleeping rough), 87% were male, the largest age groups being those aged 25–44 (46%) and 18–24 (16%). People aged 60 and over made up 7% of the total, and 16–17 year olds were 3%. When asked about experiences of institutional living 24% said they had been raised in a children's home, 46% had been in a remand centre or prison at some time and 20% said they had been an inpatient in a psychiatric hospital.

Other work on single homeless people and homeless families demonstrates that they are at increased risk of a range of diseases. Single homeless people have 2.8 times the risk of premature death compared with non-homeless people. They have 156 times the risk of death from assault or murder, 7.7 times the risk of fatal accident and 33 times the risk of suicide. Levels of mental illness are high in homeless people and there is evidence that some types of mental illness (in the absence of appropriate health and social services) leads to homelessness. Being homeless is itself a severe stressor which results in very high levels of depression and contributes to the high levels of substance abuse found in rough sleepers especially.

Getting people off the streets is one way of tackling this problem but a better way is to focus on why people become homeless. This is a complex problem but it reduces to the unsurprising fact that a person becomes homeless when he or she has a housing need but has no claim to secure housing. The stereotype of a young woman becoming pregnant so she could 'jump' the housing queue has no basis in the reality of housing need. Yet this was a principal reason cited by ministers in the former Conservative Government for drastically changing the legislation on homelessness (via the Housing Act 1996). Prior to this change certain categories of homeless people were granted statutory rights to secure permanent housing if they were accepted by a local authority as homeless (so-called 'priority need' groups). Prior to the May 1997 election no statutory rights were claimable by any group. Instead of permanent housing, those who were accepted by local authorities as homeless were given temporary accommodation and, if deemed not to have made sufficient attempts at seeking their own secure accommodation, could after one year be refused further assistance. Such people and families would not, however, appear on official statistics because they would not have been accepted as homeless. Officially accepted homelessness in Britain has increased from 63 013 in 1978 to 169 966 in 1992. These figures measure households, not persons, and exclude those who were not officially accepted, estimated at two to three times this number.

At the time of writing (June 1997) local authorities have been instructed to reinstate their former procedures regarding granting priority need status. This interim measure, though welcome, must be made a statutory requirement and form part of a coherent national housing policy.

Such a policy is overdue because evidence suggests that access to housing has been falling during the period when officially recorded homelessness has been rising. The sale of council houses and the virtual cessation of newly built council housing is one reason for this. The thrust of housing policy (1979–97) was to see home ownership as the 'natural' form of housing, other types of tenure being seen as transitional or as residual, for those unable to buy. Rather than providing 'bricks and mortar' (building new housing) the central role of government was seen as ensuring a healthy housing market. To those who could not afford home ownership, Housing Benefit (HB) was introduced so that such people could use the private rented and social (Council and Housing Association) sectors to provide their housing.

However, demand outstripped supply. Moreover, HB expenditure leapt from £200 million in 1979 to over £4 billion in 1992. This prompted a reform of HB which meant that eligibility was further restricted and levels of support were capped. Most commentators believe that these changes along with those on homelessness will prove disastrous, making more and more people and families insecure in their housing. The policy of HB has proved to be no policy at all. It has worked to deter the taking up of employment opportunities, it maintains insecurity of tenure and, in its present form, increases insecurity and fails to meet genuine need.

The health damaging effects of poor housing conditions, insecure housing and homelessness have been reported extensively in the research literature, yet housing policy, as we have seen, appeared in the years 1979–97 to be exacerbating the damage. One further illustration will prove useful in making this argument. Because of restrictions on direct government subsidies to housing associations (HAs) (introduced by the former Conservative administration) the rent charged by HAs has had to increase to 'market levels'. However, because low-income working households have severe restrictions on how much HB they may claim (the 'poverty trap') it is non-working households, who quality for full HB, who are predominantly now able to enter this type of housing. Consequently, this creates ghettos of un-employment and socially deprived households. A new form of geographical segregation has thus been created, dependent upon poverty and mediated through a misjudged housing policy.

Education

Excellent education, particularly at primary and secondary level, is a critical factor in equipping individuals with the knowledge, skills and attitudes they will require to live a healthy and fulfilling life. Moreover, educated individuals form an educated society, increasing the opportunities of all its members to enjoy the highest levels of collective well-being. Unfortunately, there is too much variation in the quality of education available to large sections of the population. The National Commission on Education report *Learning to Succeed* (1993) summarized the situation:

> A minority of academically able young people receive a good, if narrow education and, for them, provision is well suited and efficiently run. For a majority of people, education is of more variable benefit.

> ... the talents of many are not valued enough and not developed enough; and, once they start work, the same is true in terms of training. In addition, an uncomfortably large minority of young people leaving school have trouble with literacy and numeracy and seem to have benefited all too little from their education.

It is education that holds the key to unlocking inequalities in health. Intergenerational relative mobility between the social classes has not had a pronounced effect in equalizing life chances – including the chance of an excellent education – since the Second World War. In this sense the Welfare State has failed. Social mobility is not a key feature in our society. Excellent education is at present, still, largely confined to selective schools. However, we need to be clear about our definition of 'excellence'.

In the task of judging education from a public health perspective we can discern two factors. First, there seems to be a causal role for education in explaining health inequalities; second, excellent education, by its nature, forms a large component of any coherent conception of quality of life or well-being. In constructing our public health view on education these two factors share equal importance. Education at present appears to be the single most important element in achieving what upward social mobility there is, and hence allows such individuals to escape the health effects of lower social class. However, the causal role of education in setting up and maintaining personal factors which act in a health-promoting way may not necessarily rely upon upward mobility in a social class system. Even if upward social mobility is facilitated by education, this connection should not be thought of as essential for the health effects of education. For instance, in a society that was not as stratified as ours, it is quite possible (we suggest likely) that there would still be a relationship between excellent education and good health. Gough and Doyal make this case in their discussion of human needs and there is empirical support for this view (see Chapter 3).

What constitutes excellence in education? Turning this into an answerable question we need to be clear about the form, timing and content of schooling. The National Commission on Education suggested that successful schools were characterized by certain features (see Box 7.3). It is important to remember that schools cannot do everything. Parents and social and economic conditions play a large role in helping or hindering an excellent education. But it is also important to start the drive for excellence somewhere.

In terms of planning and feasibility, starting with schools is more sensible than exhorting parents or society to change. Moreover, there is ample evidence that excellence in schooling can compensate to some extent for adverse home circumstances. Education is therefore a major key to public health.

Conclusion

This chapter has examined the *HoN* from the point of view of a broader conception of those tasks that a realist health policy should engage with. The *HoN* is judged to have been a compromise, an attempted balancing of what was perceived as a practical strategy with one better grounded in the causal pathways to disease. A realist health policy is one that is based upon

---

Box 7.3: Features of a successful school

1 Strong, positive leadership by the head and senior staff

2 A good atmosphere or spirit, generated both by shared aims and values and by a physical environment that is as attractive and stimulating as possible

3 High and consistent expectations of all pupils

4 A clear and continuing focus on teaching and learning

5 Well-developed procedures for assessing how pupils are progressing

6 Participation by pupils in the life of the school

7 Rewards and incentives to encourage pupils to succeed

8 Parental involvement in children's education and in supporting the aims of the school

9 Extracurricular activities that broaden pupils' interests and experiences, expand their opportunities to success, and help to build good relationships within the school

Source: National Commission on Education Report (1993): pp. 142–3.

---

the lessons that health inequalities have to teach. The final section of this chapter outlined the divided nature of the UK and described the principal problems which connected up to produce and reproduce health inequalities. It is these divisions and others such as racism that a realist health policy must now confront.

Case study

The public health contribution to improving unequal health

The drive towards 'multi-sector' working, enshrined as one of the *HFA 2000* core values, and later much encouraged (and re-named) in the 'health alliances' approach, has turned out to have been one of the most productive of actions to reduce inequalities in health in Britain in recent years. As Sir Douglas Black remarked in 1991: '...We may be reasonably confident that there will be no simple single explanation for the association between low income and poor health ...'. He pointed out that poverty and other forms of social deprivation bring with them many disadvantages, some of which are recognized as risks to health, e.g. poor housing, over-crowding, greater liability to accidents in cramped homes. In addition, poverty also brings out other difficulties: in gaining access to health care, inadequate take-up of preventive measures, the specific risks of certain (poorly paid) occupations and greater prevalence of risky lifestyle factors, not the least of which is smoking.

Following established principles, many public health physicians have identified and analysed an increasing amount of epidemiological information about inequalities. This can range from assembling routine data about one disease area, e.g. age-adjusted rates for cancer of the cervix, stomach and lung, which are found to be greatest for people living in council housing, in people with no access to a car (a marker of relative poverty) and in manual workers, through to recognizing considerable inequalities in, say, men's health. At a more sophisticated level the work has involved carrying out a thorough assessment of health needs in a particularly deprived area of an inner city. Additional information about health needs can be obtained through the Total Systems Development (TSD) approach. This is a fully inclusive model incorporating all disciplines involved in health and social care and specifically collects users' views to help shape services.

The TSD approach develops, delivers and evaluates methods of promoting health change:

- to individuals – via one to one work

- to groups – via targeted interventions

- to geographic populations – via work in areas of high deprivation and through work with individual practices.

Having identified information (typically at a localized level), particular work can then be carried out with other agencies, e.g. local authorities or with voluntary organizations, to tackle and meet these health needs. Typical projects have included:

- meeting the health needs of homeless people by appointing a GP and/or health visitors, together with ensuring better informed health agencies who facilitate the use of preventive measures

- working with local authorities to ensure that repair action is carried out on damp houses and/or reduction of over-crowding (with emphasis also given to injury control measures)

- specific health programmes targeted at reducing health inequalities in particular population groups, e.g. multi-agency men's health networks; a multiplicity of projects tackling the health of minority ethnic communities; community safety (anti-crime) programmes attempting to reduce much fear and anxiety in, for example, older people and women in certain built-up inner city areas.

These and many other projects are often funded by health and local authorities and other agencies and must, of course, be evaluated to be of real value. Whilst we recognize that the NHS has only a part to play in the maintenance and improvement of health we suggest that health needs identification, option appraisal with partners and then implementation with evaluation are core public health tasks that can make a decisive NHS contribution to tackling disease and promoting health.

Notes

The CMO's report is published annually by HMSO. The *Health of the Nation* was published as a Consultation (Green) Paper in 1991 (cm1523) and as a White Paper in 1992 (cm1986) by HMSO. For comment on the *HoN* see, for example, John Ashton's article 'The Health of the Nation' (*BMJ* [editorial]. 1991; **302**: 1413–4); Radical Statistics Health Group 'Missing: a strategy for health of the nation' (*BMJ*. 1991; **303**: 209–302); John Gabbay 'The health of the nation' (*BMJ* [editorial]. 1992; **305**: 129–30). For a good analysis from the Henley Centre of the 'enterprise' culture and 'me' generation see Stewart Lansley's book *After the Gold Rush* (London: Century Books, 1994). The epidemiological effects of risk factor decreases are inferred from a number of sources. For the relationship between blood pressure and cardiovascular disease see, Rory Collins *et al.* 'Blood pressure, stroke, and coronary heart disease' (Parts 1 and 2.) (*Lancet*. 1990; **335**: 765–74 and 827–38). For the relationship of cholesterol and diet to coronary disease see Malcolm Law *et al.* 'Cholestrol papers' (*BMJ*. 1994; **308**: 363–80). For the survey data mentioned see, *Health Survey for England 1994* (London: HMSO, 1996). The HFA 2000 targets and strategy are in *Targets for Health For All* (WHO Regional Office for Europe: 1985). *Healthy People 2000* was published in 1990 by the

US Department of Health and Human Services, DHHS Publication No. (PHS) 91-50213. The mortality statistics are from: Drever F, Whitehead M and Roden M (1996) Current patterns and trends in male mortality by social class (based on occupation), *Population Trends* **86:** 15–20. Peter Townsend's Book *A Poor Future* (London: Lemos and Crane, 1996) contains invaluable information on poverty gained through Parliamentary questions (PQs). A B Atkinson's analysis of income inequality is in *New Inequalities* (ed., John Hills) (Cambridge: Cambridge University Press, 1996). Employment statistics are regularly published in *The Employment Gazette*, and there is an excellent analysis of atypical employment in *Social Security and Social Change* (eds, Sally Baldwin and Jane Falkingham) (London: Harvester Wheatsheaf, 1994). For job insecurity see, Nicholas Adnett's book *European Labour Markets – Analysis and Policy* (Harlow: Addison Wesley Longman, 1996). Housing and homelessness and their impact on health is covered in *Homelessness and Ill Health* (eds, Jim Connelly and June Crown) (London: Royal College of Physicians of London Working Party Report, 1994), social policy aspects of housing are covered by Paul Balchin in *Housing Policy* (London: Routledge, 1995). Housing conditions and ill-health are well covered in *Unhealthy Housing* (eds, Roger Burridge and David Ormandy) (London: E and F N Spon, 1993). The Paul Hamlyn Foundation National Commission on Education Report *Learning to Succeed* contains a wealth of statistics on the divisions within education (London: Heinemann, 1993). The Case Study refers to work by T Kelly *Total Systems Development Approach* (Huddersfield: Calderdale and Kirklees Health Authority, 1996).

8

Where now?

This book has not attempted to describe in detail the work of public health physicians; rather we have attempted to display the tasks that confront public health practice. Though doctors will remain an important group, these tasks confront the wider community of public health practitioners. The arguments for two clear tasks have formed the substance of this book:

(1) The formulation of a realist health policy, and

(2) The reform of clinical medicine.

It is our view that these tasks are interconnected (see Chapters 4 and 5), specifically that the social ideology of biomedicine constitutes a barrier to the acceptance of a socio-political analysis of health and disease, and the making of a realist health policy. We, unlike others, do not see this state of affairs as an impasse – medicine can and indeed has changed and the task is to persuade and facilitate further changes. Thus public health medicine is critical of certain aspects of biomedicine but is not critical of medicine; there is no question that a reformed medicine will be a valued social institution and profession in any possible future.

In each chapter of this book we have posed a question and, we hope, have formulated a public health perspective in our answers. The institutional history of public health medicine in the UK has offered numerous threats and opportunities for effective practice. By tracing this history (Chapter 1) we hope to have demonstrated that though a *unifying theory* of public health practice has eluded adoption, there has been considerable progress in creating professional consensus over the problems to be confronted and the tools and skills needed by practitioners. Certainly, this consensus among public health practitioners (a larger group than public health physicians) is being actively shaped by the evidence that social, economic and political factors have a causal influence on health and disease.

The task of using this new knowledge in shaping clinical discussion is centrally important for public health. Specifically, in the UK, moving the NHS agenda away from 'cure' to an 'effective cure' and 'efficient and appropriate care' service is inextricably tied to the public health visions of Thomas McKeown (Chapter 2) and Archie Cochrane (Chapter 5). However, re-structuring should not be viewed as a parochial concern; health systems worldwide are currently in need of radical reconstruction. Public health must assist in this needed change by education and persuasion. Education of the public is not simply one of many options, it is the only option. An informed public will, within a democratic society, demand restructuring of its social institutions to protect and promote health.

Thus our public health perspective on the reform of health systems, and clinical medicine, sees change plainly as a political task. In this, it echoes Rudolf Virchow's nineteenth century insight and asks professional politic-ians, power-brokers and anyone else with influence to recognize that dis-ease and health are largely created by our own actions. Unlike biomedicine, however, public health locates the blame primarily at the door of our social organization rather than our lifestyles.

That lifestyles are freely chosen is a basic assumption of libertarians. On this assumption it is quite possible, even necessary, to ascribe blame to indi-viduals for causing their ill health. That things are not so simple has been argued (Chapter 3) and forms one premise for an alternative strategy for health (Chapters 4 and 7). This strategy we have variously called socio-political or, more succinctly, a realist strategy. Chapter 7 outlines the types of problem such a strategy should confront in this nation. Making a realist health strategy happen, however, is the major problem. Social justice, after all, is hardly a new concept and political parties have different view points regarding what is just. If public health understanding and practice leaves things as they are it will have failed its purpose. It must confront counter arguments head on.

To libertarians whatever was legally obtained in the past becomes indi-vidual property and the just society would protect these individual property rights above all other claims. To socialists like Gerry Cohen in his book *Equality and the Right to Self Ownership* there are, ultimately, no compelling reasons why people should give up their property rights; any change towards equality must be because people choose or are tolerant of the change. Andrew Glyn and David Miliband in their book *Paying for Inequality*, how-ever, provide details of the costs which are borne by all of us, allowing the argument that it is these social costs which make more equality a rational choice, one even driven by self-interest. Brian Barry, as we saw (Chapter 5), identifies justice as impartiality; here the question is 'How would I feel if I were in his (or her) situation?', it derives its ethical force from our natural ability as human beings to identify ourselves with the plight of others. To this imaginative act the new knowledge about inequalities as a cause of disease must be assimilated.

Consequently, social justice questions become health questions and political discourse becomes health discourse. The grounds for inequalities must, if they are to be informed, justify the health consequences of inequalities. As we have discussed (Chapters 5 and 7), it is no longer sufficient for the health sector to be seen as the most rational place for tackling or preventing ill health. A realist health policy cannot be confined to the health sector – it simply misses the point to attempt this. So what is necessary?

At a minimum, the political conversation that society keeps going with itself must expand its horizons. Biomedicine has enabled politics to disengage with the human needs that will maintain and promote health. To this end, then, biomedicine (as a social ideology) must be disarmed. As we suggested, it is possible that this transformation will be triggered by the inadequacy of biomedicine's paradigm. This paradigm is not delivering its promised bounty (Chapter 6) and there is increasing confidence in rival camps. However, as Kuhn suggested, it may take a generation to die out for the new paradigm to become established, because persuasion, even given the better argument, rarely makes converts. Public health practitioners are an important part of this paradigm shift, working with others both within clinical medicine and outside it, for a changed view.

The kind of society that seriously values health will need to reassess its fundamental, that is taken-for-granted, beliefs. It is not a matter of 'going against nature', for example, to suggest that economic analysis that sees the free market as its exemplar is not only empirically a nonsense but makes no theoretical sense either. Jon Mulberg, in his book *The Social Limits To Economic Theory*, shows that classical and neo-classical economic theory is riddled with unresolved problems. The eclipse of planning that is seen by some as the major achievement of libertarian theory, is shown to be greatly overstated. It is possible to plan for economic progress and for an economy in the service of the needs of human beings.

The narrowness of orthodox economics forms an important strand in the work of Amartya Sen. In particular, Sen argues for an expansion of the conceptual techniques of welfare economics and a return to a political economy viewpoint, where politics is part of economics and, consequently, ethics is also reintroduced. In terms of our discussion on rationing health care these developments supply a theoretical ground for our approach. Two scenarios were described: a possible future 'cure' and 'care' service whose emergence is dependent on a realistic assessment of the limits of clinical medicine, and a current scenario where the factors of technology, demographics and, above all, expectations create a demand for health care that outstrips supply. In managing the current situation one technique of health economics, marginal programme budgeting (MPB), was singled out for its practical usefulness.

It was made clear, however, that rationing decisions cannot be made on grounds of 'economic rationality' alone. Values and questions regarding justice pervade rationing decisions. Yet it is too simple to say that this problem can be tackled by recourse to the choices of the 'public'. Whilst, we suggest, a public voice is required for legitimate choices to be made, these choices must be moderated within a shared ethical framework. A short account of a true story will illustrate why.

In 1962, Dr Belding Scribner of the University of Washington Medical School came up with a practical device for connecting patients with chronic renal failure to a kidney machine. These patients underwent this new treatment, known as dialysis, for eight hours three times per week. The dialysis treatment worked like their kidney should have, cleansing their blood of impurities and allowing them to survive what would otherwise be a terminal condition. The kidney machines, however, were in very short supply and there were far more people who would benefit from dialysis treatment compared to what was available. This posed a clear cut need to ration the treatment.

The Seattle Medical Society confronted this problem by establishing a committee of seven citizens, none of whom had any special qualifications. Initially, this committee comprised a lawyer, a church minister, a housewife, a union leader, a state government official, a banker and a surgeon. All eligible patients were referred to this committee for the life-or-death decision, *who should receive treatment*?

It is a matter of record that things did not really go to plan. A report in *Life Magazine* by Shana Alexander described how committee members used standards such as whether a man was married with children as conferring priority over single men and women and childless couples. 'Public service', seen as churchgoing or activity in voluntary projects, was similarly given priority. The committee saw anyone with a mental disability or a criminal record as 'deviant' and rejected their claim for treatment. Consequently, the charge was that this committee of the public was using what many would consider to be narrow middle-class based criteria for evaluating terminally ill patients. The concept of 'public service' was questioned by commentators. As an illustration, it was said that the great American literary figure Thoreau would have little chance of qualifying for treatment. Thoreau's 'deviancy' was his quest to understand nature by choosing to live alone in Walden wood: 'I went into the wood to live deliberately', he wrote. The *UCLA Law Review* wrote: 'The Pacific Northwest is no place for a Henry David Thoreau with bad kidneys'.

There is, then, nothing especially ethical in devolving rationing decisions to committees of 'the public'. The decisions that groups make, whether they are experts or not, must be subject to ethical criteria. As we have argued effectiveness of the treatment together with its opportunity cost are relevant criteria within an ethical framework, as is the existing distribution of resources. The application of Rawlsian principles of justice may mean that less treatment goes to those who have more resources, but, as we argued, a Rawlsian approach confined to the health sector would leave the societal mechanisms that produce unjust shares in the first place largely untouched. In terms of our current predicament it appears that the only possibility of avoiding rationing is to establish our first scenario through the means of the second, current, scenario. Whilst this transformation occurs, however, rationing choices will be, and indeed are being, made. Public input into these choices, via for example, *citizen juries* or *citizen panels*, within an ethical framework, currently provides the most appropriate method for rationing decisions.

The alternative to the explicit establishment of rationing is its continued and concealed existence within professional and organizational contexts. Would such deliberations today produce decisions unlike those of the 1962 Seattle Committee? Our opinion is that given similar resource constraints, today's decisions would not differ in any substantial detail from those made in 1962. Though it is difficult to do, hard choices do have to be made in current health systems, the real issue is how to make decisions that are just.

Before we close this book it is worth noting the inadequacy of a public health practice which is not political, that is, which does not contain a view or theory of what is good and right for people. Certainly the social sciences have debated whether a political neutrality is possible or desirable but we wish to go further. Our view is that public health must necessarily work to establish a set of views that are irreducibly political. Neutrality is not an option. To argue this we may follow the philosopher Charles Taylor's methods in his essay *Neutrality in Political Science* (1967). By 'political science', Taylor intends any 'policy' science, i.e. any applied social science.

Taylor begins by noting that a strict empiricism is not possible, facts are not simply before us, we select observable events and by applying causal explanations attempt to make sense of the world. Thus an explanation provides us with a framework for ordering and correlating the observed facts. But by accepting a framework as a useful means we unavoidably also accept 'the values the framework secretes'. Taylor demonstrates this by discussing Lipset's theory of democracy, we can demonstrate it by following up the inequalities in health facts and seeing what sort of values are unavoidably revealed by our explanatory framework.

In brief, as we have seen, the evidence points to social, economic and political factors as having a causal influence on the risks of disease or health. Those who are in the higher social classes are less likely to suffer morbidity and premature death compared with those in the lower social classes. Now if we accept the fact that health is better than disease – as, surely, all rational humans are able to do – then health is valued as a *good*. It is something we would commend and choose for ourselves. We would, then, rationally wish to bring about health rather than disease on our own behalf. But, for a number of reasons, diseases of others can interfere with our own health, so I (you) ought to wish that everyone can attain health. The reasons we wish there to be general good health can be construed in economic or ethical terms. Communicable diseases, for example, do not just affect me but may be passed on to you – this is an example of an *externality*. Moreover, my suffering a disease may reduce your enjoyment of your own good health; consequently it becomes rational for you to care about my health as well as about your own.

The upshot of this is that social, economic and political factors that increase the risk of disease are to be considered *bad*, and the policies which result in this state are *wrong*. A good policy should either eliminate inequalities or minimize their effects. Of course, it is possible to produce arguments against this conclusion. Taylor shows these arguments are of two types, *overriding* and *undermining* arguments.

An overriding argument would acknowledge the validity of these conclusions but would produce an argument which would attempt to trump it by being deemed to be more important. For example, equalizing incomes may well infringe on individual property rights and this may be used to counter the arguments for equality that have gained their *moral* force by our evaluating ill-health as bad. However, the framework that produces this overriding value (property rights) is a different framework. If we wish to improve health then our original framework prescribes what is good and what is bad. This demonstrates that even if political discourse integrated the lessons of inequalities in health there would still be scope for political arguments (what framework matters most?). We suggest, however, that even so, inequality would be more difficult to justify and the arguments from property rights would be more difficult to sustain.

An undermining argument, however, claims that the values we have derived from the framework are inaccurate or non-existent. So equality, the value derived from the inequalities in the health framework, is said to be not connected in the way we have shown it to be connected. But as Taylor demonstrates, an undermining argument can only be sustained as the value expression of a different explanatory framework. It leaves the original framework intact but poses (in this case) a weak alternative. For inequality to be the value the framework would have to show how inequality improved health. As this is not in fact the case the undermining argument fails.

What is the use of this discussion? First, it demonstrates that in the social sciences at least *you can get an 'ought' from an 'is'* – a result said to be impossible in much classical philosophy, where a moral prescription cannot be derived from a description of the facts. For human life, however, a description of the facts inescapably carries a moral prescription. Recourse to a claim of 'neutrality' is not a possibility. Second, specifically, it shows that public health analyses cannot possibly be merely descriptive. In short, public health, informed by the facts regarding health inequalities, is inescapably political.

Notes

For Rudolf Virchow's project see George Rosen's *History of Public Health* (New York: MD Publications, 1958). Gerry Cohen's book *Equality and the Right of Self Ownership* (Cambridge: Cambridge University Press, 1995) deals with the arguments against proceduralist theories of justice and rights, exemplified by Robert Nozick's work. Andrew Glyn and David Miliband's *Paying for Inequality* is co-published by the left-of-centre think tank, the Institute for Public Policy Research (London: IPPR/Rivers Oram Press, 1994). Jon Mulberg's *The Social Limits To Economic Theory* (London: Routledge, 1995) is a critique of the 'naturalism' of neo-classical economic theory. The story of the Seattle Medical Committee is given by David J Rothman in his article *Rationing Life* in the *New York Review of Books*, March 5, 1992. Charles Taylor's article *Neutrality in Political Science* is in Ryan A (ed.) *The Philosophy of Social Explanation* (Oxford: OUP, 1990).

Index